Pain Management

Editors

PERRY G. FINE
MICHAEL A. ASHBURN

ANESTHESIOLOGY CLINICS

www.anesthesiology.theclinics.com

Consulting Editor
LEE A. FLEISHER

June 2016 • Volume 34 • Number 2

ELSEVIER

1600 John F. Kennedy Boulevard • Suite 1800 • Philadelphia, Pennsylvania, 19103-2899

http://www.theclinics.com

ANESTHESIOLOGY CLINICS Volume 34, Number 2
June 2016 ISSN 1932-2275, ISBN-13: 978-0-323-44607-5

Editor: Patrick Manley
Developmental Editor: Kristen Helm

Anesthesiology Clinics (ISSN 1932-2275) is published quarterly by Elsevier Inc., 360 Park Avenue South, New York, NY 10010-1710. Months of issue are March, June, September, and December. Periodicals postage paid at New York, NY and at additional mailing offices. Subscription prices are $100.00 per year (US student/resident), $330.00 per year (US individuals), $400.00 per year (Canadian individuals), $596.00 per year (US institutions), $753.00 per year (Canadian institutions), $225.00 per year (Canadian and foreign student/resident), $455.00 per year (foreign individuals), and $753.00 per year (foreign institutions). To receive student and resident rate, orders must be accompanied by name of affiliated institution, date of term, and the *signature* of program/residency coordinator on institutions letterhead. Orders will be billed at individual rate until proof of status is received. Foreign air speed delivery is included in all *Clinics'* subscription prices. All prices are subject to change without notice. POSTMASTER: Send address changes to *Anesthesiology Clinics,* Elsevier Health Sciences Division, Subscription Customer Service, 3251 Riverport Lane, Maryland Heights, MO 63043. Customer Service (orders, claims, online, change of address): Elsevier Health Sciences Division, Subscription Customer Service, 3251 Riverport Lane, Maryland Heights, MO 63043. **Tel:1-800-654-2452 (U.S. and Canada); 314-447-8871 (outside U.S. and Canada). Fax: 314-447-8029. E-mail: journalscustomerservice-usa@elsevier.com (for print support); journalsonlinesupport-usa@elsevier.com (for online support).**

Reprints. For copies of 100 or more of articles in this publication, please contact the Commercial Reprints Department, Elsevier Inc., 360 Park Avenue South, New York, NY 10010-1710. Tel.: 212-633-3874; Fax: 212-633-3820; E-mail: reprints@elsevier.com.

Anesthesiology Clinics, is also published in Spanish by McGraw-Hill Inter-americana Editores S. A., P.O. Box 5-237, 06500 Mexico D. F., Mexico.

Anesthesiology Clinics, is covered in *MEDLINE/PubMed (Index Medicus), Current Contents/Clinical Medicine, Excerpta Medica, ISI/BIOMED*, and *Chemical Abstracts*.

Printed in the United States of America.

Contributors

CONSULTING EDITOR

LEE A. FLEISHER, MD, FACC, FAHA
Robert D. Dripps Professor and Chair of Anesthesiology and Critical Care, Professor of Medicine, Perelman School of Medicine Health System, University of Pennsylvania, Philadelphia, Pennsylvania

EDITORS

PERRY G. FINE, MD
Professor of Anesthesiology, Department of Anesthesiology, Pain Research Center, University of Utah School of Medicine, Salt Lake City, Utah

MICHAEL A. ASHBURN, MD, MPH
Professor of Anesthesiology and Critical Care Senior Fellow, Department of Anesthesiology and Critical Care, Penn Pain Medicine Center, University of Pennsylvania, Philadelphia, Pennsylvania

AUTHORS

IGNACIO J. BADIOLA, MD
Instructor of Anesthesiology, Pain Management and Critical Care, Department of Anesthesiology and Critical Care, Perelman School of Medicine, University of Pennsylvania; Penn Pain Medicine Center, Philadelphia, Pennsylvania

JAIME L. BARATTA, MD
Assistant Professor, Department of Anesthesiology, Sidney Kimmel Medical College, Thomas Jefferson University, Philadelphia, Pennsylvania

SHANE E. BROGAN, MB BCh
Associate Professor, Department of Anesthesiology, University of Utah School of Medicine, Salt Lake City, Utah

MARTIN D. CHEATLE, PhD
Center for Studies of Addiction, Perelman School of Medicine, University of Pennsylvania, Philadelphia, Pennsylvania; Reading Health System, West Reading, Pennsylvania

LARA DHINGRA, PhD
MJHS Institute for Innovation in Palliative Care, New York, New York

KATHRYN N. DUENSING, JD
Researcher and Policy Analyst, American Academy of Pain Management, Sonora, California

SIMMIE FOSTER, MD, PhD
Kirby Center for Neurobiology, Boston, Massachusetts

ROLLIN M. GALLAGHER, MD, MPH
National Program Director for Pain Management, Veterans Health Administration, Michael Crescenz VA Medical Center; Clinical Professor of Psychiatry and Anesthesiology, Director for Pain Policy Research and Primary Care, Penn Pain Medicine, University of Pennsylvania, Philadelphia, Pennsylvania

AARON M. GILSON, MS, MSSW, PhD
Research Program Manager/Senior Scientist, Pain and Policy Studies Group, Carbone Cancer Center, University of Wisconsin, Madison, Wisconsin

SUSAN D. HORN, PhD
Adjunct Professor, Department of Population Health Sciences, Health System Innovation and Research Division, University of Utah School of Medicine, Salt Lake City, Utah

CHARLES E. INTURRISI, PhD
Professor of Pharmacology, Department of Pharmacology, Weill Cornell Medical College, New York, New York

MATTHEW LESNESKI, MD
RA Pain Services, Mount Laurel, New Jersey

SEAN C. MACKEY, MD, PhD
Chief, Division of Pain Medicine; Redlich Professor, Department of Anesthesiology, Perioperative and Pain Medicine; Director, Stanford Systems Neuroscience and Pain Lab (SNAPL); Neurosciences and Neurology, by courtesy, Stanford University School of Medicine, Palo Alto, California

KATHERINE T. MARTUCCI, PhD
Postdoctoral Research Fellow, Division of Pain Medicine, Department of Anesthesiology, Perioperative and Pain Medicine, Stanford University School of Medicine, Palo Alto, California

NEEL MEHTA, MD
Assistant Professor of Anesthesiology, Department of Anesthesiology; Medical Director, Weill Cornell Pain Medicine, Weill Cornell Medical College, New York, New York

SERGEY M. MOTOV, MD
Department of Emergency Medicine, Maimonides Medical Center, Brooklyn, New York

LEWIS S. NELSON, MD
New York University School of Medicine, New York, New York

AARON PINKETT, BS
Center for Studies of Addiction, Perelman School of Medicine, University of Pennsylvania, Philadelphia, Pennsylvania

DAVID QU, MD
Highpoint Pain and Rehabilitation Physicians P.C., Chalfont, Pennsylvania

ERIC S. SCHWENK, MD
Assistant Professor, Department of Anesthesiology, Sidney Kimmel Medical College, Thomas Jefferson University, Philadelphia, Pennsylvania

JILL E. SINDT, MD
Assistant Professor, Department of Anesthesiology, University of Utah School of Medicine, Salt Lake City, Utah

ROBERT K. TWILLMAN, PhD
Executive Director, American Academy of Pain Management, Sonora, California

EUGENE R. VISCUSI, MD
Professor, Department of Anesthesiology, Sidney Kimmel Medical College, Thomas Jefferson University, Philadelphia, Pennsylvania

LYNN R. WEBSTER, MD
Vice President of Scientific Affairs, PRA Health Sciences, Salt Lake City, Utah

JOHN T. WENZEL, MD
Clinical Instructor, Department of Anesthesiology, Sidney Kimmel Medical College, Thomas Jefferson University, Philadelphia, Pennsylvania

LISA R. WITKIN, MD
Assistant Professor of Anesthesiology, Department of Anesthesiology, Weill Cornell Pain Medicine, Weill Cornell Medical College, New York, New York

Contents

Foreword: Chronic Pain and Its Treatment in an Era of Increased Scrutiny   xi

Lee A. Fleisher

Preface: Pain Management   xiii

Perry G. Fine and Michael A. Ashburn

Imaging Pain   255

Katherine T. Martucci and Sean C. Mackey

> The challenges and understanding of acute and chronic pain have been illuminated through the advancement of central neuroimaging. Through neuroimaging research, new technology and findings have allowed us to identify and understand the neural mechanisms contributing to chronic pain. Several regions of the brain are known to be of particular importance for the maintenance and amplification of chronic pain, and this knowledge provides novel targets for future research and treatment. This article reviews neuroimaging for the study of chronic pain, and in particular, the rapidly advancing and popular research tools of structural and functional MRI.

Advanced Concepts and Controversies in Emergency Department Pain Management   271

Sergey M. Motov and Lewis S. Nelson

> Pain is the most common complaint for which patients come to the emergency department (ED). Emergency physicians are responsible for pain relief in a timely, efficient, and safe manner in the ED. The improvement in our understanding of the neurobiology of pain has balanced the utilization of nonopioid and opioid analgesia, and simultaneously has led to more rational and safer opioid prescribing practices. This article reviews advances in pain management in the ED for patients with acute and chronic pain as well as describes several newer strategies and controversies.

Managing Opioid-Tolerant Patients in the Perioperative Surgical Home   287

John T. Wenzel, Eric S. Schwenk, Jaime L. Baratta, and Eugene R. Viscusi

> Management of acute postoperative pain is important to decrease perioperative morbidity and improve patient satisfaction. Opioids are associated with potential adverse events that may lead to significant risk. Uncontrolled pain is a risk factor in the transformation of acute pain to chronic pain. Balancing these issues can be especially challenging in opioid-tolerant patients undergoing surgery, for whom rapidly escalating opioid doses in an effort to control pain can be associated with increased complications. In the perioperative surgical home model, anesthesiologists are positioned to coordinate a comprehensive perioperative analgesic plan that begins with the preoperative assessment and continues through discharge.

Can Chronic Pain Be Prevented?   303

Ignacio J. Badiola

All chronic pain begins at some discrete point in time. Significant strides in the understanding of mechanisms and risk factors associated with the transition from a new, or acute, pain experience to a chronic pain condition have been made over the past 20 years. These insights provide the hope of one day being able to modify or even halt this pathophysiologic progression. This article reviews some of the current knowledge of this transition as well as the evidence currently available to best prevent and treat it using persistent surgical pain as a model.

Interventional Treatments of Cancer Pain   317

Jill E. Sindt and Shane E. Brogan

Pain is a significant burden for patients with cancer and is particularly prevalent among those with advanced cancer. Appropriate interventional cancer pain therapies complement conventional pain management by reducing the need for systemic opioid therapy and its associated toxicity; however, these therapies are often underutilized. This article reviews techniques, indications, complications, and outcomes of the most common interventional approaches for the management of cancer-related pain. These approaches include intrathecal drug delivery, vertebral augmentation, neurolysis of the celiac, superior hypogastric and ganglion impar plexus', image-guided tumor ablation, and other less commonly performed but potentially beneficial interventions.

Chronic Pain and the Opioid Conundrum   341

Lynn R. Webster

Opioids prescribed for chronic cancer and noncancer pain have been embroiled in public policy debates as to effectiveness and potential for contributing to society's problem with misuse, addiction, and overdose mortality. The conundrum of opioid prescribing is to determine who will most likely benefit from opioids and how medical practitioners may safely provide chronic opioid therapy, while also identifying patients who are unlikely to benefit or could divert illicit pharmaceuticals into society. Risk assessment and monitoring are essential to meet the standard of care, as is compliance with federal controlled substances law as well as state regulations.

Advancing the Pain Agenda in the Veteran Population   357

Rollin M. Gallagher

The Veterans Health Administration (VHA) provides medical care for Veterans after leaving the military. The combination of multiple deployments and battlefield exposures to physical and psychological trauma results in a higher prevalence and complexity of chronic pain in Veterans than in the general public. The VHA and the Department of Defense work together to develop a single standard of stepped pain management appropriate for all settings from moment of injury or disease onset. This article describes the education, academic detailing, and clinical programs and policies that are transforming pain care in the VHA.

Assessing and Managing Sleep Disturbance in Patients with Chronic Pain 379

Martin D. Cheatle, Simmie Foster, Aaron Pinkett, Matthew Lesneski, David Qu, and Lara Dhingra

Chronic pain is associated with symptoms that may impair a patient's quality of life, including emotional distress, fatigue, and sleep disturbance. There is a high prevalence of concomitant pain and sleep disturbance. Studies support the hypothesis that sleep and pain have a bidirectional and reciprocal relationship. Clinicians who manage patients with chronic pain often focus on interventions that relieve pain, and assessing and treating sleep disturbance are secondary or not addressed. This article reviews the literature on pain and co-occurring sleep disturbance, describes the assessment of sleep disturbance, and outlines nonpharmacologic and pharmacologic treatment strategies to improve sleep in patients with chronic pain.

Using Chronic Pain Outcomes Data to Improve Outcomes 395

Neel Mehta, Charles E. Inturrisi, Susan D. Horn, and Lisa R. Witkin

Standardization of care that is derived from analysis of outcomes data can lead to improvements in quality and efficiency of care. The outcomes data should be validated, standardized, and integrated into ongoing patient care with minimal burden on the patient and health care team. This article describes the organization and workflow of a chronic pain clinic registry designed to collect and analyze patient data for quality improvement and dissemination. Future efforts in using mobile technology and integrating patient-reported outcome data in the electronic health records have the potential to offer new and improved models of comprehensive pain management.

State Policies Regulating the Practice of Pain Management: Statutes, Rules, and Guidelines That Shape Pain Care 409

Robert K. Twillman, Aaron M. Gilson, and Kathryn N. Duensing

In response to increased awareness of prescription opioid misuse, abuse, addiction, diversion, and overdose, states have promulgated a large number of public policies intended to regulate the practice of pain medicine. Nearly every state now has at least 1 type of policy; others only provide recommendations to physicians. This article reviews the existing policies and extracts specific provisions within each of them. Although there are many similarities across policies, unique features are found in some and are specifically reviewed. This review can serve as a quick reference for policymakers and as a guide for researchers interested in the impacts of such policies.

Index 425

FORTHCOMING ISSUES

September 2016
Advances in Neuroscience in Anesthesia and Critical Care
W. Andrew Kofke, *Editor*

December 2016
Medically Complex Patients
Stanley H. Rosenbaum and
Robert B. Schonberger, *Editors*

March 2017
Obstetric Anesthesia
Robert R.Gaiser and Onyi Onuoha,
Editors

RECENT ISSUES

March 2016
Preoperative Evaluation
Debra Domino Pulley and Deborah C.
Richman, *Editors*

December 2015
Value-Based Care
Lee A. Fleisher, *Editor*

September 2015
Geriatric Anesthesia
Charles H. Brown IV and Mark D. Neuman,
Editors

THE CLINICS ARE AVAILABLE ONLINE!
Access your subscription at:
www.theclinics.com

Foreword

Chronic Pain and Its Treatment in an Era of Increased Scrutiny

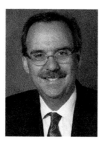

Lee A. Fleisher, MD, FACC, FAHA
Consulting Editor

Chronic pain is a major health care problem that has significant impact on an individual's quality of life and significant economic impact from both costs of treatment and loss of productivity. In addition, our ability to treat chronic pain has variable effectiveness, and many of the interventions have not been studied using rigorous methods such as randomized controlled trials using validated outcome instruments. There are many vulnerable populations with respect to chronic pain. Veterans are particularly at risk given that many have sustained significant physical injuries and there are overlaying mental health challenges. When patients with chronic pain undergo surgery, management can be very complex, and most physicians outside of those trained in chronic pain management are ill prepared to treat these patients. Finally, we have an epidemic of prescription opioid abuse that is just being recognized, and state and federal agencies and legislatures are just beginning to develop programs to help reduce the problem while trying to determine best interventions.

Drs Fine and Ashburn represent an outstanding team of authors addressing this issue. Perry G. Fine, MD is Professor of Anesthesiology at the University of Utah and is on the faculty of the Pain Research Center and an Attending Physician in the Pain Management Center. He serves on the Board of Directors, is Immediate Past President of the American Academy of Pain Medicine, and represents the Academy on the Steering Committee of the Pain Care Coalition. Michael A. Ashburn, MD, MPH, MBA is Professor of Anesthesiology and Critical Care at the University of Pennsylvania and Director of the Penn Pain Management Center. He was past President of the American Pain Society and a past member of the Commonwealth of Pennsylvania Prescription Drug Abuse Task Force. Both have subspecialty certification in pain

Anesthesiology Clin 34 (2016) xi–xii
http://dx.doi.org/10.1016/j.anclin.2016.03.002
1932-2275/16/$ – see front matter © 2016 Published by Elsevier Inc.

anesthesiology.theclinics.com

medicine and Hospice and Palliative Care. The issue provides a guide to the current state of the art, science, and policy around the complex issues of the treatment of chronic pain.

Lee A. Fleisher, MD, FACC, FAHA
Perelman School of Medicine Health System
University of Pennsylvania
3400 Spruce Street, Dulles 680
Philadelphia, PA 19104, USA

E-mail address:
Lee.Fleisher@uphs.upenn.edu

Preface

Pain Management

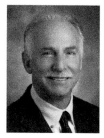 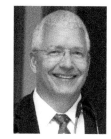

Perry G. Fine, MD   Michael A. Ashburn, MD, MPH
Editors

The formative years of pain medicine as a distinct field of study, practice, and research transpired during the last half of the twentieth century. It was not an easy "childhood," with fits and starts of growth and development over many years, with little formal recognition by accrediting bodies, payers, or policy-makers. But finally, due to a convergence of demographic shifts (most notably our aging society), cultural shifts, scientific advances, and societal demands, there has been a coming of age in this second decade of the twenty-first century. The "coming-out party" was marked by the Institute of Medicine of the National Academy of Sciences publication, "Relieving Pain in America: A Blueprint for Transforming Prevention, Care, Education, and Research." This publication led to the recently released National Pain Strategy by the National Institutes of Health, wherein six key areas are to be addressed:

1. Determination of just how big and how severe chronic pain is as a public health issue.
2. Better emphasis on prevention of acute and chronic pain.
3. Improvement in the quality of pain care and reduction of barriers to underserved populations at risk for pain.
4. How to make sure that access to optimal pain management is available to all.
5. More education and training for the people who deliver care.
6. Creation of a national pain awareness campaign and promotion of safe medication use by patients.

In order for any of these objectives to be realized—no less make a "dent" in the large-scale national public health and economic problems manifest in the unnecessary suffering and huge financial toll due to inadequately treated pain—medical practitioners of all disciplines, but especially anesthesiologists, who have unique skills to prevent, diagnose, and manage myriad pain conditions, need to stay current in this burgeoning field. This issue of *Anesthesiology Clinics* affords this opportunity.

Anesthesiology Clin 34 (2016) xiii–xiv
http://dx.doi.org/10.1016/j.anclin.2016.03.001
1932-2275/16/$ – see front matter © 2016 Published by Elsevier Inc.

As long-time friends and colleagues, we worked together for many years during an earlier phase of our careers, along with several other faculty members within the Department of Anesthesiology at the University of Utah, developing both the Acute Pain Management Service (inpatient acute care) and the Interdisciplinary Chronic Pain Management Center (inpatient, outpatient cancer, and noncancer chronic pain care). Along the way, we valued the opportunity provided to us every few years to edit compendia of contemporary topics in pain management. This occurred due to the commitment of an outstanding mentor, Dr Ted Stanley, to bring internationally recognized experts to Salt Lake City, as speakers at nationally attended annual meetings. And, every few years, the topic of pain management would take its turn in the rotation—and we gladly accepted the task of editing the content of those talks into book form. This became the means by which clinicians, educators, and researchers could rapidly update themselves through a convenient summary of "what's new and developing."

Time passed; resources for such gatherings and publications dried up, but the need is still there. And so it is with great joy, and a sense of reunion, that we come together again as guest editors of this topical issue. We are grateful to Dr Lee Fleisher for the honor of this assignment, and the opportunity he has provided us to join forces yet again, on behalf of our guest authors, *Anesthesiology Clinics* readership, and most importantly, the patients who will benefit from your continued self-education in this field.

With limited space, we have been highly selective in topics represented, with an effort to showcase updates and reviews in the areas of pain-related basic science and neurobiology, applied clinical practice embracing several different types of care settings, and current policy issues. We hope you find these articles to be compelling reading, relevant to your respective practice, and most of all, useful in some way for the very next patient who puts their hopes for relief and a better life in your hands.

Perry G. Fine, MD
Department of Anesthesiology
Pain Research Center
University of Utah School of Medicine
Suite 200, 615 Arapeen Drive
Salt Lake City, UT 84109, USA

Michael A. Ashburn, MD, MPH
Department of Anesthesiology and Critical Care, Penn Pain Medicine Center
University of Pennsylvania
1840 South Street
Philadelphia, PA 19146, USA

E-mail addresses:
perry.fine@hsc.utah.edu (P.G. Fine)
michael.ashburn@uphs.upenn.edu (M.A. Ashburn)

Imaging Pain

Katherine T. Martucci, PhD, Sean C. Mackey, MD, PhD*

KEYWORDS

- Chronic pain • Neuroimaging • MRI • Resting-state networks • MVPA
- Brain-based therapies

KEY POINTS

- No single region within the central nervous system is responsible for chronic pain; altered brain structure and function occurs across many regions of the brain, brainstem, and spinal cord.
- Resting-state functional MRI (fMRI) has revealed multiregional alterations in brain function within various resting-state networks, including the salience, executive control, and default-mode networks.
- Multivariate pattern analysis (MVPA) is a new and powerful technology that allows for a whole-brain approach to identify altered brain structure and function in chronic pain. MVPA may ultimately help to develop brain-based objective biomarkers of pain and achieve the goal of precision pain management.
- Researchers are now using neuroimaging to identify brain targets for novel and effective treatments for chronic pain, such as transcranial magnetic stimulation, real-time fMRI, and other neuroimaging-based therapies.

INTRODUCTION

Chronic pain affects more than 100 million adults and accounts for approximately $600 billion annually in medical costs and lost productivity.[1]

The complex neural mechanisms that occur to amplify and maintain chronic pain are poorly understood. Neuroimaging pain research holds great promise for the development of new and effective treatments through advancing our understanding of these complex mechanisms.

Neuroimaging research findings show that chronic pain is different from acute pain. Chronic pain can become a disease in its own right that occurs following initial injury, which then progresses to a chronic state within the central nervous system (CNS). Although other body systems are also involved in the initiation and maintenance of

Conflict of Interest Statement: Authors have no conflicts of interest to declare.
Funding Sources: K99 DA040154, K24 DA29262 and the Redlich Pain Research Endowment.
Department of Anesthesiology, Perioperative and Pain Medicine, Division of Pain Medicine, Stanford Systems Neuroscience and Pain Lab (SNAPL), 1070 Arastradero Road, Suite 200, MC 5596, Palo Alto, CA 94304-1345, USA
* Corresponding author. Department of Anesthesiology, Perioperative, and Pain Medicine, Division of Pain Medicine, 1070 Arastradero Road, Suite 200, MC 5596, Palo Alto, CA 94304-1345.
E-mail address: smackey@stanford.edu

Anesthesiology Clin 34 (2016) 255–269
http://dx.doi.org/10.1016/j.anclin.2016.01.001
1932-2275/16/$ – see front matter

chronic pain,[2] neuroimaging has allowed for increased understanding of how the CNS is involved in chronic pain.

Types of neuroimaging used to study chronic pain
- PET
- Electroencephalography (EEG)
- Magnetoencephalography (MEG)
- Single-photon emission computed tomography (SPECT/CT)
- MRI

Examples of chronic pain conditions studied using neuroimaging
- Chronic low back pain (cLBP)[3]
- Fibromyalgia (FM)[4]
- Osteoarthritis (OA)[5]
- Complex regional pain syndrome (CRPS)[6]
- Phantom limb pain, chronic migraine[7]
- Chronic pelvic pain (CPP)[8,9]
- Peripheral neuropathy (PN)[10]

In addition to advancing the study of chronic pain, the evolution of neuroimaging technology has opened a window to the brain that allows us a more complete understanding of the basic physiologic and pathophysiologic mechanisms of pain signal processing and the related subjective experience of pain itself.

Examples of neuroimaging research of pain processing
- Acute pain in healthy volunteers[11]
- Acute pain in animals[12]
- Animal models of chronic pain[13]

Several experiential factors influence the experience of pain. Neuroimaging has allowed for the study of how these factors interact with and impact pain perception by studying related changes in brain activity.

Examples of pain modulatory factors studied using neuroimaging
- Attention[14]
- Anticipation[15]
- Empathy[16]
- Placebo[17]
- Effects of meditation[18]
- Fear/anxiety[19]
- Reward[20]

The present review focuses specifically on the use of neuroimaging, specifically the most widely used neuroimaging technology of MRI, and observed CNS changes in various chronic pain conditions (**Box 1**) As used here in this review, we refer to "neuroimaging" as meaning imaging of the spinal cord, brainstem, and brain. Neuroimaging of peripheral nerves is beyond the scope of this review.

ANATOMIC AND FUNCTIONAL SUBSTRATES
Basic Sequence of Mechanisms and Structures Involved in Pain Processing

1. Noxious stimuli trigger signals in the peripheral nerves. Peripheral nerves that relay nociceptive information include the following:
   - A-delta nerve fibers: These fibers transmit "first-pain" signals, the pricking, sharp sensations felt immediately after a stimulus.

> **Box 1**
> **MRI protocols**
>
> MRI is a widely used neuroimaging tool for the study of chronic pain. It combines a strong magnetic field with radiofrequency pulses to display high spatial-resolution structural images. Multiple imaging protocols using MRI have been developed and allow for measurement of changes in brain structure and activity.
>
> Voxel-based morphometry, cortical thickness analysis: measures the density and distribution of gray matter.
>
> Diffusion tensor imaging, functional anisotropy: measures the density and distribution of white matter.
>
> Functional MRI (fMRI): indirect measure of brain activity based on changes in blood oxygenation level (referred to as the BOLD signal)[21]
>
> Magnetic resonance spectroscopy: measures relative concentrations of metabolites[22]
>
> Arterial spin labeling fMRI: measures changes in global and regional blood flow by using magnetically labeled protons in the blood as an endogenous tracer[23]
>
> Neuroimaging protocols can collect data from patients with chronic pain when they are at rest, performing various tasks, or undergoing interventions and procedures.
>
> *Examples of Neuroimaging Nonrest Conditions*
>
> - Application of physical stimuli
>   - Heat pain
>   - Pressure
>   - Movement of the body (eg, limb) to evoke pain
> - Tasks
>   - Showing emotion-evoking images
>   - Working memory tasks
>   - Decision-making tasks
>
> *Data from* Refs.[21–23]

- C fibers: These fibers transmit "second-pain" signals, the dull, aching, throbbing pain felt 1 to 2 seconds after a stimulus.[24]
2. The peripheral nerve fibers synapse in the dorsal horn of the spinal cord.
3. Interneurons are responsible for inhibitory/excitatory modulation at the level of the spinal cord.
4. Secondary spinal projection neurons transmit nociceptive information to the brainstem regions, including the rostral ventral medulla and periaqueductal gray (PAG).
5. Nociceptive information is further modulated in the brainstem and then relayed to the thalamus.
6. The nociceptive signals are transmitted from the thalamus to the cortex where they are interpreted as pain.
7. Several cortical regions are involved in pain processing, including the primary somatosensory cortex, secondary somatosensory cortex, insular cortex, prefrontal cortex, and motor cortex (for review, see Ref.[25]).

In chronic pain, these systems are thought to be upregulated, causing a state of "central sensitization."[26] Central sensitization is the result of the following:

- Inflammation and sensitized receptors in the skin causing abnormal or increased nociceptive signals from peripheral nerves
- Lack of inhibition and/or increased excitation within the spinal cord, brainstem, and/or cortex

Neuroimaging allows for noninvasive measurement of altered activity in the spinal cord, brainstem, and brain, where pain modulation and central sensitization occur and contribute to chronic pain.[27] Historically, neuroimaging researchers have focused their efforts on finding key brain regions that have altered structure and activity in individuals with chronic pain. The identification of specific brain regions implicated in mechanisms that support ongoing chronic pain may allow future targets for therapy.

Several key brain regions are known to play major roles in chronic pain. These regions most commonly function as regions of sensory and motor processing, affective and emotional aspects of pain, and high-order cortical processing and integration.

IMAGING FINDINGS
Regional Changes in Brain Structure

Numerous research studies have investigated brain structure in individuals with chronic pain typically using methods of voxel-based morphology (VBM)[28] and cortical thickness analysis.[29] Increased and decreased cortical thickness and gray matter density occur among several chronic pain conditions, including cLBP,[3,30] fibromyalgia,[31] temporomandibular disorders (TMD),[20] CRPS,[6] migraine,[32] and in chronic visceral pain, such as irritable bowel syndrome (IBS).[33] Newer research studies have investigated changes in gray matter among multiple types of chronic pain, such as CRPS, knee OA, and cLBP.[34] Together, these studies show that key areas of gray matter differences are most often within the following:

- Somatosensory and motor cortex
- Insular cortex
- Subcortical regions including the thalamus and basal ganglia
- Parietal cortex
- Prefrontal cortex
- Amygdala and hippocampus

Changes in gray matter are most commonly observed as decreases in regional gray matter density. These decreases in gray matter density may be associated with increased age-related gray matter atrophy.[35] However, several studies show both regional increases and decreases in gray matter density.[20] Thus, the primary cause of these changes is unclear. It is also unknown whether these observations represent preexisting differences in brain structure; in other words, that may predispose persons to chronic pain. Alternatively, the changes in gray matter density may result from the presence of chronic pain, for example, due to ongoing stress of the pain experience.

It is also unclear whether these changes may be *functionally* linked to the maintenance of chronic pain. Further, differences in gray matter structure may be specifically due to chronic pain, or may result from the many comorbid conditions or other factors often observed in conjunction with chronic pain, such as depression, sleep disturbance, or medication use. As an example of this, in a meta-analysis of structural brain changes in patients with FM, depression scores accounted for most of the changes in gray matter structure.[36] Nonetheless, gray matter changes are likely not only due to depression, because these changes also have been observed in patients with cLBP experiencing very minimal levels of comorbid depression.[3]

Changes in white matter structure are also commonly observed in neuroimaging research studies of chronic pain. These changes represent the structural integrity of connections between brain regions. Diffusion tensor imaging (DTI) and fractional anisotropy are the primary technologies used to measure white matter structure within the brain. Differences in white matter structure have been observed among several chronic pain states, including TMD,[37] IBS,[38] and CPP.[39]

Newer research has measured changes in gray matter and white matter simultaneously. These studies have been conducted in patients with CRPS[40] and FM[41,42] and allow for increased understanding of the relationships between gray and white matter structural changes in chronic pain.

Regional Changes in Brain Function

Altered brain activity has been detected across multiple chronic pain syndromes. Most of the brain regions that demonstrate functional changes overlap with regions of observed structural change.[43] Neuroimaging research studies often measure brain activity in individuals with chronic pain in response to painful stimulation,[44] during emotional or cognitive tasks,[45] in response to stress,[46] or while patients continuously rate their ongoing pain.[47]

Similar to acute pain processing, multiple brain regions appear to play a functional role in chronic pain.[48] Several key regions in the CNS consistently demonstrate altered function in chronic pain across numerous neuroimaging research studies, described as follows.

Primary somatosensory cortex and posterior insular cortex:
- Regions typically associated with intensity coding of pain
- Altered activity (typically increased) in response to noxious stimulation
- Observed in cLBP, FM, CPP, and CRPS[49]
- Suggest altered intensity processing of pain in chronic pain

Secondary somatosensory cortex (SII):
- Region of higher-order sensory processing and integration
- Structural and functional alterations observed in this region[50]

Primary motor cortex, premotor cortex, and supplementary motor areas:
- Regions of motor processing and preparation of movement
- Structural and functional alterations have been observed in in CPP[9,51]
- Implicated in chronic pain due to close overlap of brain sensory and motor processes

Cerebellum:
- Functional changes often reported yet minimally discussed in the literature
- May be related to altered sensory-motor and emotional processing in the presence of chronic pain[52]

Prefrontal cortex (PFC):
- Includes the ventromedial PFC, dorsolateral PFC, and orbitofrontal PFC[53]
- Higher-order regions of cognitive processing and cognitive inhibition of pain
- Regions mediate the relationship between cognitive processes and chronic pain (for example see Ref.[54])

Parietal cortex:
- Includes the temporo-parietal junction, precuneus, and posterior cingulate cortex

- Regions are involved in introspection, mind wandering, and self-referential thought processes[55]
- Functional changes in chronic pain may reflect increased integration of thought processes with pain experience

Anterior insular cortex[56] and anterior cingulate cortex[57]:
- Regions related to the affective aspects of pain processing (such as the level of unpleasantness, negative context)
- Altered function in chronic pain[58]

Amygdala[59] and hippocampus[60]:
- Regions involved in emotion, fear, and memory processes
- Functional alterations related to psychological aspects of chronic pain, including altered fear and emotional processing
- Scale-based correlations of altered emotion processing with altered brain structure and function
- Alterations due to general changes in limbic and memory networks because fear avoidance (of movement) is not responsible for these changes[61]

Subcortical, midbrain, and brainstem regions:
- Functional alterations suggest altered brain circuits and modulation of nociceptive information
- Thalamic lesions implicated in central pain[62] and altered thalamic activity in other chronic pain states as well
- Basal ganglia[63]
- Midbrain regions, including the ventral tegmental area,[64,65] altered mechanisms of reward, punishment, and dopamine function

Brainstem regions:
- PAG[66] may signify disrupted regulatory control of pain[67]
- Because of its small size, highly complex structure, and the multifunctional heterogeneity of the brainstem, thus far there is limited study within this region

Spinal cord:
- Altered activity observed using electrophysiology, typically in animal models of chronic pain
- MRI of the cervical spinal cord in healthy individuals[68,69]
- Technology is evolving, and in the future may be useful for the study of chronic pain[70]

Network-Based Changes in Brain Function

Resting-state functional MRI (fMRI) focuses on relationships of activity across multiple brain regions, or "networks." Correlated activity between regions within a network indicates that regions are functionally connected.[71] Resting-state fMRI is used to collect information about the natural state of brain activity because the data are collected while participants are at rest. It is therefore ideal for patients with chronic pain because no additional sensory or cognitive stimulation is necessary. Functional connectivity is measured as the correlation of low-frequency oscillations in neural activity among brain regions. Differences in functional connectivity implicate altered resting-state brain activity in individuals with chronic pain.[72] Several resting-state networks show increased or decreased functional connectivity in chronic pain.[73] These include the default-mode networks (DMN),[74] regions more active at rest; salience and executive control networks, regions more active during sensory stimulation or tasks; and sensory-motor networks, regions related to sensory and motor processes. Altered DMN function in chronic pain states has been demonstrated also using arterial spin labeling fMRI.[75]

In cLBP, decreased functional connectivity within the DMN has been observed, in particular among regions of the medial PFC, posterior cingulate cortex, and amygdala.[76] In FM, increased functional connectivity has been observed within the DMN and executive attention network.[77] Greater connectivity between the DMN and insular cortex has also been observed in FM, which suggests the relationship between these regions is altered in FM.[77] Similar alterations in the relationship between the insular cortex and other cortical regions have been observed in other studies of FM as well.[78] Alterations in the low-frequency fluctuations within the primary somatosensory cortex, supplementary motor area, dorsolateral prefrontal cortex, and amygdala also have been observed in chronic pain.[79] Decreased functional connectivity within the DMN and increased functional connectivity within sensory, motor, and other pain-processing regions occurs in CRPS.[80] In CPP, altered resting-state activity occurs in sensory-motor regions[81] and within the DMN.[82] Additional research has demonstrated that altered functional connectivity of the brainstem,[83] basal ganglia,[84] and regions of the frontal and temporal cortices[85] occur in chronic migraine. Similar alterations in resting-state activity have been shown to occur in diabetic neuropathic pain.[86]

Multivariate Analysis of Neuroimaging Data

Multivariate pattern analysis (MVPA) uses machine-learning technology and is ideal for analysis of large neuroimaging data sets (for review see Ref.[87]). MVPA also can be used to identify signature patterns of changes in brain structure and function that may represent subgroups of patients with chronic pain. Additionally, MVPA can function as a prediction tool. Once a chronic pain signature pattern has been identified, data from a single individual can be classified (eg, as belonging to a healthy person or person with chronic pain) based on its similarity to the originally identified signature pattern of chronic pain.[88] MVPA technology has been used to identify acute pain–related changes in healthy human volunteers,[11] and can be used to differentiate patients with chronic pain from healthy volunteers based on brain structure.[3,9]

MVPA technology may make neuroimaging useful as a diagnostic tool. It may provide the ability to predict an individual patient's prognosis and to define the appropriate therapy based on an individual patient's brain structure and activity patterns (**Fig. 1**). Overall, MVPA is a powerful tool that may greatly advance the clinical utility of neuroimaging for individuals with chronic pain and may help us to achieve the goal of precision pain medicine.

Longitudinal Limitations of Chronic Pain Neuroimaging Research

Most neuroimaging studies of chronic pain to date are cross-sectional. Therefore, causation of observed functional and structural changes cannot be inferred from most neuroimaging research. Longitudinal studies would allow tracking chronic pain from its onset and potentially causative information. Recently, some longitudinal investigations have been conducted, in cLBP[89] and IBS.[90] Changes in white matter structure have been shown paralleling the transition from subacute to cLBP.[91] Some brain changes are even reversed after treatment with effective therapies,[92] for example, psychological therapy.[93] Thus, although CNS alterations are abundant in chronic pain states, these alterations are likely not permanent. The use of appropriate and effective therapies may reduce chronic pain, and while doing so, restore normal brain structure and function (**Box 2**).

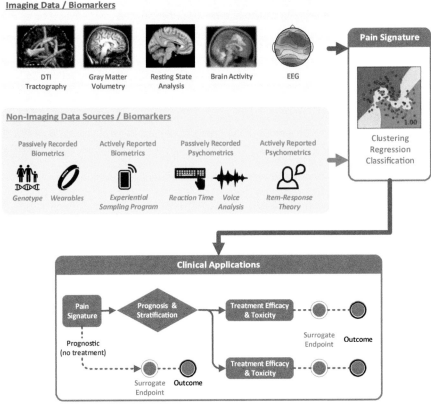

Fig. 1. Schematic of data sources and clinical applications related to identification of pain signature patterns imaging data can provide large sources of detailed and objective biomarkers for pain (*top, gray box*). Various sources of imaging biomarkers include (1) structural abnormalities measured with MRI (eg, DTI of white matter tractography; gray matter volumetry), (2) functional differences measured with fMRI (eg, resting-state fMRI networks and functional connectivity between brain regions; brain activity in response to evoked stimulation or during a task), and (3) functional differences measured with non-MRI modalities, such as EEG. Nonimaging data sources can provide additional objective biomarkers (*middle, green box*). These include, for example, genotype information, biometrics from wearable technology (eg, actigraphy), actively reported biometrics (eg, via handheld devices for recording patients' symptoms throughout the day), psychometrics including reaction time tests and voice analysis (eg, to measure emotional states, such as depression or anxiety) and actively reported psychometrics (ie, demographic, psychological, and clinical questionnaires). The identified biomarkers from both imaging and nonimaging sources can be combined as input for an MVPA. The MVPA uses clustering, regression, and/or classification technology and is capable of identifying the most meaningful biomarkers to provide a multivariable signature pattern of pain (*right, red box*). The MVPA-derived pain signature can then be used in a variety of clinical applications (*bottom, red box*). Starting as a complex prognostic measure, the pain signature could provide the basis for stratification of an individual to a specific treatment program ("Prognosis & Stratification"). Surrogate endpoints, follow-up measurements after treatment, could be used to evaluate the treatment as effective or noneffective for the individual patient. Ultimately, the final outcome measures would indicate the pain signature's prognostic sensitivity and specificity. Alternatively, as a more traditional clinical course of action ("Prognostic [no treatment]"), the pain signature could be used simply as a diagnostic (for clinical or legal purposes) or to predict a patient's prognosis over time regardless of treatment. (*Courtesy of* Ming-Chih Kao, PhD, MD, Palo Alto, CA.)

Box 2
Neuroimaging-based therapies

Several real-time neurofeedback studies have been conducted for chronic pain.[94,95] Additional research studies and clinical trials are still needed.

Deep brain stimulation and motor cortex stimulation are invasive therapies. They are therefore used only for use in very severe, intractable cases of chronic pain. Newer tools are being developed to better select patients who will most likely benefit.[96] Current techniques use adaptive models[97] and target brain regions that have the potential to activate multiple downstream effects.[98]

Transcranial magnetic stimulation (TMS) is a noninvasive intervention to reduce symptoms of chronic pain. Clinical trials of TMS demonstrate reduced pain for days to weeks after treatment.[99] Current TMS research objectives are to identify better brain region targets and delivery specifications (such as parameters and treatment frequency).

Novel advancements for the future use of neuroimaging in chronic pain–related therapy include the development of brain-computer interfaces using electrocorticography and visual feedback. Visual feedback may be a beneficial therapy for phantom limb pain.[100]

Data from Refs.[94–100]

SUMMARY

Neuroimaging research has opened a window to the brain. Evidence of altered brain structure and function has been found across most chronic pain conditions. Common chronic pain conditions of cLBP, FM, neuropathic pain, and TMD have been frequently investigated using neuroimaging. Now that neuroimaging has identified tangible alterations in brain structure and function, chronic pain is less often thought of with skepticism as a mere psychological representation. Numerous neuroimaging studies have repeatedly demonstrated extensively altered brain structure and function across multiple types of chronic pain.

A large amount of overlapping evidence has been collected, all of which suggests that altered brain mechanisms greatly contribute to chronic pain. Neuroimaging research has identified multiple brain regions involved in processes of pain, sensory, motor, cognitive, motivational, memory, emotion, and fear that are related to chronic pain. A challenge for clinical care of chronic pain remains the individual variability in the pain experience among patients, with each patient's condition being different from another's. Further research and future advances in neuroimaging technology may clarify how brain mechanisms are involved in chronic pain and allow for the development of novel neuroimaging-based therapies for chronic pain.

ACKNOWLEDGMENTS

Special thanks to Dr Ming-Chih Kao for designing **Fig. 1**.

REFERENCES

1. IOM. Relieving pain in America: a blueprint for transforming prevention, care, education, and research. Washington, DC: IOM; 2011.
2. Mackey SC. Central neuroimaging of pain. J Pain 2013;14(4):328–31.
3. Ung H, Brown JE, Johnson KA, et al. Multivariate classification of structural MRI data detects chronic low back pain. Cereb Cortex 2014;24(4):1037–44.
4. Staud R. Brain imaging in fibromyalgia syndrome. Clin Exp Rheumatol 2011; 29(6 Suppl 69):S109–17.

5. Howard MA, Sanders D, Krause K, et al. Alterations in resting-state regional cerebral blood flow demonstrate ongoing pain in osteoarthritis: an arterial spin-labeled magnetic resonance imaging study. Arthritis Rheum 2012;64(12): 3936–46.

6. Barad MJ, Ueno T, Younger J, et al. Complex regional pain syndrome is associated with structural abnormalities in pain-related regions of the human brain. J Pain 2014;15(2):197–203.

7. Chiapparini L, Ferraro S, Grazzi L, et al. Neuroimaging in chronic migraine. Neurol Sci 2010;31(Suppl 1):S19–22.

8. Farmer MA, Chanda ML, Parks EL, et al. Brain functional and anatomical changes in chronic prostatitis/chronic pelvic pain syndrome. J Urol 2011; 186(1):117–24.

9. Bagarinao E, Johnson KA, Martucci KT, et al. Preliminary structural MRI based brain classification of chronic pelvic pain: a MAPP network study. Pain 2014; 155(12):2502–9.

10. Moisset X, Bouhassira D. Brain imaging of neuropathic pain. Neuroimage 2007; 37(Suppl 1):S80–8.

11. Brown JE, Chatterjee N, Younger J, et al. Towards a physiology-based measure of pain: patterns of human brain activity distinguish painful from non-painful thermal stimulation. PLoS One 2011;6(9):e24124.

12. Jeffrey-Gauthier R, Guillemot JP, Piche M. Neurovascular coupling during nociceptive processing in the primary somatosensory cortex of the rat. Pain 2013; 154(8):1434–41.

13. Thompson SJ, Millecamps M, Aliaga A, et al. Metabolic brain activity suggestive of persistent pain in a rat model of neuropathic pain. Neuroimage 2014;91: 344–52.

14. Lawrence JM, Hoeft F, Sheau KE, et al. Strategy-dependent dissociation of the neural correlates involved in pain modulation. Anesthesiology 2011;115(4): 844–51.

15. Fairhurst M, Wiech K, Dunckley P, et al. Anticipatory brainstem activity predicts neural processing of pain in humans. Pain 2007;128(1–2):101–10.

16. Ochsner KN, Zaki J, Hanelin J, et al. Your pain or mine? Common and distinct neural systems supporting the perception of pain in self and others. Soc Cogn Affect Neurosci 2008;3(2):144–60.

17. Watson A, El-Deredy W, Iannetti GD, et al. Placebo conditioning and placebo analgesia modulate a common brain network during pain anticipation and perception. Pain 2009;145(1–2):24–30.

18. Zeidan F, Martucci KT, Kraft RA, et al. Brain mechanisms supporting the modulation of pain by mindfulness meditation. J Neurosci 2011;31(14):5540–8.

19. Ochsner KN, Ludlow DH, Knierim K, et al. Neural correlates of individual differences in pain-related fear and anxiety. Pain 2006;120(1–2):69–77.

20. Younger JW, Shen YF, Goddard G, et al. Chronic myofascial temporomandibular pain is associated with neural abnormalities in the trigeminal and limbic systems. Pain 2010;149(2):222–8.

21. Logothetis NK. The underpinnings of the BOLD functional magnetic resonance imaging signal. J Neurosci 2003;23(10):3963–71.

22. Widerstrom-Noga E, Pattany PM, Cruz-Almeida Y, et al. Metabolite concentrations in the anterior cingulate cortex predict high neuropathic pain impact after spinal cord injury. Pain 2013;154(2):204–12.

23. Williams DS. Quantitative perfusion imaging using arterial spin labeling. Methods Mol Med 2006;124:151–73.

24. Price DD, Hu JW, Dubner R, et al. Peripheral suppression of first pain and central summation of second pain evoked by noxious heat pulses. Pain 1977; 3(1):57–68.
25. Willis WD, Westlund KN. Neuroanatomy of the pain system and of the pathways that modulate pain. J Clin Neurophysiol 1997;14(1):2–31.
26. Latremoliere A, Woolf CJ. Central sensitization: a generator of pain hypersensitivity by central neural plasticity. J Pain 2009;10(9):895–926.
27. Woolf CJ. Central sensitization: implications for the diagnosis and treatment of pain. Pain 2011;152(3 Suppl):S2–15.
28. Ashburner J, Friston KJ. Voxel-based morphometry–the methods. Neuroimage 2000;11(6 Pt 1):805–21.
29. Chung MK, Worsley KJ, Robbins S, et al. Deformation-based surface morphometry applied to gray matter deformation. Neuroimage 2003;18(2):198–213.
30. Schmidt-Wilcke T, Leinisch E, Ganssbauer S, et al. Affective components and intensity of pain correlate with structural differences in gray matter in chronic back pain patients. Pain 2006;125(1–2):89–97.
31. Kuchinad A, Schweinhardt P, Seminowicz DA, et al. Accelerated brain gray matter loss in fibromyalgia patients: premature aging of the brain? J Neurosci 2007; 27(15):4004–7.
32. Schmidt-Wilcke T, Ganssbauer S, Neuner T, et al. Subtle grey matter changes between migraine patients and healthy controls. Cephalalgia 2008;28(1):1–4.
33. Davis KD, Pope G, Chen J, et al. Cortical thinning in IBS: implications for homeostatic, attention, and pain processing. Neurology 2008;70(2):153–4.
34. Baliki MN, Schnitzer TJ, Bauer WR, et al. Brain morphological signatures for chronic pain. PLoS One 2011;6(10):e26010.
35. May A. Chronic pain may change the structure of the brain. Pain 2008; 137(1):7–15.
36. Smallwood RF, Laird AR, Ramage AE, et al. Structural brain anomalies and chronic pain: a quantitative meta-analysis of gray matter volume. J Pain 2013; 14(7):663–75.
37. Moayedi M, Weissman-Fogel I, Salomons TV, et al. White matter brain and trigeminal nerve abnormalities in temporomandibular disorder. Pain 2012; 153(7):1467–77.
38. Ellingson BM, Mayer E, Harris RJ, et al. Diffusion tensor imaging detects microstructural reorganization in the brain associated with chronic irritable bowel syndrome. Pain 2013;154(9):1528–41.
39. Farmer MA, Huang L, Martucci K, et al. Brain white matter abnormalities in female interstitial cystitis/bladder pain syndrome: a MAPP network neuroimaging study. J Urol 2015;194(1):118–26.
40. Geha PY, Baliki MN, Harden RN, et al. The brain in chronic CRPS pain: abnormal gray-white matter interactions in emotional and autonomic regions. Neuron 2008;60(4):570–81.
41. Lutz J, Jager L, De Quervain D, et al. White and gray matter abnormalities in the brain of patients with fibromyalgia: a diffusion-tensor and volumetric imaging study. Arthritis Rheum 2008;58(12):3960–9.
42. Luerding R, Weigand T, Bogdahn U, et al. Working memory performance is correlated with local brain morphology in the medial frontal and anterior cingulate cortex in fibromyalgia patients: structural correlates of pain-cognition interaction. Brain 2008;131(Pt 12):3222–31.

43. Jensen KB, Srinivasan P, Spaeth R, et al. Overlapping structural and functional brain changes in patients with long-term exposure to fibromyalgia pain. Arthritis Rheum 2013;65(12):3293–303.

44. Derbyshire SW, Jones AK, Creed F, et al. Cerebral responses to noxious thermal stimulation in chronic low back pain patients and normal controls. Neuroimage 2002;16(1):158–68.

45. Glass JM, Williams DA, Fernandez-Sanchez ML, et al. Executive function in chronic pain patients and healthy controls: different cortical activation during response inhibition in fibromyalgia. J Pain 2011;12(12):1219–29.

46. Vachon-Presseau E, Martel MO, Roy M, et al. Acute stress contributes to individual differences in pain and pain-related brain activity in healthy and chronic pain patients. J Neurosci 2013;33(16):6826–33.

47. Baliki MN, Chialvo DR, Geha PY, et al. Chronic pain and the emotional brain: specific brain activity associated with spontaneous fluctuations of intensity of chronic back pain. J Neurosci 2006;26(47):12165–73.

48. Apkarian AV, Bushnell MC, Treede RD, et al. Human brain mechanisms of pain perception and regulation in health and disease. Eur J Pain 2005;9(4):463–84.

49. Vartiainen N, Kirveskari E, Kallio-Laine K, et al. Cortical reorganization in primary somatosensory cortex in patients with unilateral chronic pain. J Pain 2009;10(8):854–9.

50. Rodriguez-Raecke R, Ihle K, Ritter C, et al. Neuronal differences between chronic low back pain and depression regarding long-term habituation to pain. Eur J Pain 2014;18(5):701–11.

51. Kutch JJ, Yani MS, Asavasopon S, et al. Altered resting state neuromotor connectivity in men with chronic prostatitis/chronic pelvic pain syndrome: a MAPP: research network neuroimaging study. Neuroimage Clin 2015;8:493–502.

52. Moulton EA, Elman I, Pendse G, et al. Aversion-related circuitry in the cerebellum: responses to noxious heat and unpleasant images. J Neurosci 2011;31(10):3795–804.

53. Bechara A, Damasio H, Damasio AR. Emotion, decision making and the orbito-frontal cortex. Cereb Cortex 2000;10(3):295–307.

54. Weissman-Fogel I, Moayedi M, Tenenbaum HC, et al. Abnormal cortical activity in patients with temporomandibular disorder evoked by cognitive and emotional tasks. Pain 2011;152(2):384–96.

55. Kucyi A, Salomons TV, Davis KD. Mind wandering away from pain dynamically engages antinociceptive and default mode brain networks. Proc Natl Acad Sci U S A 2013;110(46):18692–7.

56. Gu X, Gao Z, Wang X, et al. Anterior insular cortex is necessary for empathetic pain perception. Brain 2012;135(Pt 9):2726–35.

57. Rainville P, Duncan GH, Price DD, et al. Pain affect encoded in human anterior cingulate but not somatosensory cortex. Science 1997;277(5328):968–71.

58. Noll-Hussong M, Otti A, Wohlschlaeger AM, et al. Neural correlates of deficits in pain-related affective meaning construction in patients with chronic pain disorder. Psychosom Med 2013;75(2):124–36.

59. Simons LE, Moulton EA, Linnman C, et al. The human amygdala and pain: evidence from neuroimaging. Hum Brain Mapp 2014;35(2):527–38.

60. Aoki Y, Inokuchi R, Suwa H. Reduced N-acetylaspartate in the hippocampus in patients with fibromyalgia: a meta-analysis. Psychiatry Res 2013;213(3):242–8.

61. Barke A, Baudewig J, Schmidt-Samoa C, et al. Neural correlates of fear of movement in high and low fear-avoidant chronic low back pain patients: an event-related fMRI study. Pain 2012;153(3):540–52.
62. Nandi D, Liu X, Joint C, et al. Thalamic field potentials during deep brain stimulation of periventricular gray in chronic pain. Pain 2002;97(1–2):47–51.
63. Baliki MN, Geha PY, Fields HL, et al. Predicting value of pain and analgesia: nucleus accumbens response to noxious stimuli changes in the presence of chronic pain. Neuron 2010;66(1):149–60.
64. Loggia ML, Berna C, Kim J, et al. Disrupted brain circuitry for pain-related reward/punishment in fibromyalgia. Arthritis Rheum 2014;66(1):203–12.
65. Wood PB. Stress and dopamine: implications for the pathophysiology of chronic widespread pain. Med Hypotheses 2004;62(3):420–4.
66. Berman SM, Naliboff BD, Suyenobu B, et al. Reduced brainstem inhibition during anticipated pelvic visceral pain correlates with enhanced brain response to the visceral stimulus in women with irritable bowel syndrome. J Neurosci 2008; 28(2):349–59.
67. Heinricher MM, Tavares I, Leith JL, et al. Descending control of nociception: specificity, recruitment and plasticity. Brain Res Rev 2009;60(1):214–25.
68. Nash P, Wiley K, Brown J, et al. Functional magnetic resonance imaging identifies somatotopic organization of nociception in the human spinal cord. Pain 2013;154(6):776–81.
69. Summers PE, Ferraro D, Duzzi D, et al. A quantitative comparison of BOLD fMRI responses to noxious and innocuous stimuli in the human spinal cord. Neuroimage 2010;50(4):1408–15.
70. Summers PE, Iannetti GD, Porro CA. Functional exploration of the human spinal cord during voluntary movement and somatosensory stimulation. Magn Reson Imaging 2010;28(8):1216–24.
71. Fox MD, Snyder AZ, Vincent JL, et al. The human brain is intrinsically organized into dynamic, anticorrelated functional networks. Proc Natl Acad Sci U S A 2005; 102(27):9673–8.
72. Fox MD, Raichle ME. Spontaneous fluctuations in brain activity observed with functional magnetic resonance imaging. Nat Rev Neurosci 2007;8(9):700–11.
73. Smith SM, Fox PT, Miller KL, et al. Correspondence of the brain's functional architecture during activation and rest. Proc Natl Acad Sci U S A 2009; 106(31):13040–5.
74. Greicius MD, Krasnow B, Reiss AL, et al. Functional connectivity in the resting brain: a network analysis of the default mode hypothesis. Proc Natl Acad Sci U S A 2003;100(1):253–8.
75. Loggia ML, Kim J, Gollub RL, et al. Default mode network connectivity encodes clinical pain: an arterial spin labeling study. Pain 2013;154(1):24–33.
76. Baliki MN, Geha PY, Apkarian AV, et al. Beyond feeling: chronic pain hurts the brain, disrupting the default-mode network dynamics. J Neurosci 2008;28(6): 1398–403.
77. Napadow V, Lacount L, Park K, et al. Intrinsic brain connectivity in fibromyalgia is associated with chronic pain intensity. Arthritis Rheum 2010;62(8):2545–55.
78. Cifre I, Sitges C, Fraiman D, et al. Disrupted functional connectivity of the pain network in fibromyalgia. Psychosom Med 2012;74(1):55–62.
79. Kim JY, Kim SH, Seo J, et al. Increased power spectral density in resting-state pain-related brain networks in fibromyalgia. Pain 2013;154(9):1792–7.
80. Bolwerk A, Seifert F, Maihofner C. Altered resting-state functional connectivity in complex regional pain syndrome. J Pain 2013;14(10):1107–15.e8.

81. Kilpatrick LA, Kutch JJ, Tillisch K, et al. Alterations in resting state oscillations and connectivity in sensory and motor networks in women with interstitial cystitis/painful bladder syndrome. J Urol 2014;192(3):947–55.

82. Martucci KT, Shirer WR, Bagarinao E, et al. The posterior medial cortex in urologic chronic pelvic pain syndrome: detachment from default mode network-a resting-state study from the MAPP Research Network. Pain 2015; 156(9):1755–64.

83. Mainero C, Boshyan J, Hadjikhani N. Altered functional magnetic resonance imaging resting-state connectivity in periaqueductal gray networks in migraine. Ann Neurol 2011;70(5):838–45.

84. Yuan K, Zhao L, Cheng P, et al. Altered structure and resting-state functional connectivity of the basal ganglia in migraine patients without aura. J Pain 2013;14(8):836–44.

85. Schwedt TJ, Larson-Prior L, Coalson RS, et al. Allodynia and descending pain modulation in migraine: a resting state functional connectivity analysis. Pain Med 2014;15(1):154–65.

86. Cauda F, D'agata F, Sacco K, et al. Altered resting state attentional networks in diabetic neuropathic pain. J Neurol Neurosurg Psychiatry 2010;81(7):806–11.

87. Orru G, Pettersson-Yeo W, Marquand AF, et al. Using support vector machine to identify imaging biomarkers of neurological and psychiatric disease: a critical review. Neurosci Biobehav Rev 2012;36(4):1140–52.

88. Iuculano T, Rosenberg-Lee M, Supekar K, et al. Brain organization underlying superior mathematical abilities in children with autism. Biol Psychiatry 2014; 75(3):223–30.

89. Hashmi JA, Baliki MN, Huang L, et al. Shape shifting pain: chronification of back pain shifts brain representation from nociceptive to emotional circuits. Brain 2013;136(Pt 9):2751–68.

90. Naliboff BD, Berman S, Suyenobu B, et al. Longitudinal change in perceptual and brain activation response to visceral stimuli in irritable bowel syndrome patients. Gastroenterology 2006;131(2):352–65.

91. Mansour AR, Baliki MN, Huang L, et al. Brain white matter structural properties predict transition to chronic pain. Pain 2013;154(10):2160–8.

92. Seminowicz DA, Wideman TH, Naso L, et al. Effective treatment of chronic low back pain in humans reverses abnormal brain anatomy and function. J Neurosci 2011;31(20):7540–50.

93. Jensen KB, Kosek E, Wicksell R, et al. Cognitive Behavioral Therapy increases pain-evoked activation of the prefrontal cortex in patients with fibromyalgia. Pain 2012;153(7):1495–503.

94. Decharms RC, Maeda F, Glover GH, et al. Control over brain activation and pain learned by using real-time functional MRI. Proc Natl Acad Sci U S A 2005; 102(51):18626–31.

95. Chapin H, Bagarinao E, Mackey S. Real-time fMRI applied to pain management. Neurosci Lett 2012;520(2):174–81.

96. Baron R, Backonja MM, Eldridge P, et al. Refractory Chronic Pain Screening Tool (RCPST): a feasibility study to assess practicality and validity of identifying potential neurostimulation candidates. Pain Med 2014;15(2):281–91.

97. Schultz DM, Webster L, Kosek P, et al. Sensor-driven position-adaptive spinal cord stimulation for chronic pain. Pain Physician 2012;15(1):1–12.

98. Garcia-Larrea L, Peyron R. Motor cortex stimulation for neuropathic pain: from phenomenology to mechanisms. Neuroimage 2007;37(Suppl 1):S71–9.

99. Lefaucheur JP, Hatem S, Nineb A, et al. Somatotopic organization of the analgesic effects of motor cortex rTMS in neuropathic pain. Neurology 2006;67(11): 1998–2004.

100. Walter A, Naros N, Roth A, et al. A brain-computer interface for chronic pain patients using epidural ECoG and visual feedback. Proceedings of the 2012 IEEE 12th International Conference on Bioinformatics & Bioengineering (BIBE), Larnaca, Cyprus, November 11–13, 2012.

Advanced Concepts and Controversies in Emergency Department Pain Management

Sergey M. Motov, MD[a],*, Lewis S. Nelson, MD[b]

KEYWORDS

- Acute pain • Chronic pain • Emergency department • Pain management • Opioids
- Nonopioid analgesics

KEY POINTS

- The key to successful parenteral opioid analgesia is the titration of these analgesics regardless of the initial dosing regimen.
- The greatest limitation to the use of intravenous (IV) versus oral acetaminophen is the nearly 100-fold cost differential, which is likely not justified by any marginal improvement in pain relief.
- The use of IV subdissociative dose of ketamine administered either alone or in combination with opioids is effective for the treatment of acute pain; however, it is associated with relatively high rates of minor, short-lived adverse side effects.
- Channels/enzymes/receptors targeted analgesia allows for a broader utilization of synergistic combinations of nonopioid analgesia and more refined and judicious use of opioids.
- The ideal path for safe and effective chronic pain management focuses on rigorous evaluation of the risk of opioids abuse, misuse, and safety, and on engagement and effective counseling on the risks and benefits of all analgesics.

INTRODUCTION

Pain is the most common complaint for which patients come to the emergency department (ED), with a prevalence of 45% to 75%.[1] Pain managed in the ED may be acute and self-limited or chronic, and emergency physicians (EPs) have had to develop expertise in the management of a broad spectrum of acute and chronic painful conditions. Because poorly managed pain may cause significant behavioral, physiologic,

[a] Department of Emergency Medicine, Maimonides Medical Center, 4802 Tenth Avenue, Brooklyn, NY 11219, USA; [b] New York University School of Medicine, 455 First Avenue, New York, NY, USA
* Corresponding author.
E-mail address: smotov@maimonidesmed.org

Anesthesiology Clin 34 (2016) 271–285
http://dx.doi.org/10.1016/j.anclin.2016.01.006   **anesthesiology.theclinics.com**

and social disturbances, EPs have historically been encouraged to liberally use anal-gesics, in particular opioids, for pain, with the admonition that failure to do so will lead to subpar care and "oligoanalgesia."[2] Simultaneously, advocacy for attention to pain control with resultant increased and more widespread use of opioids in patients with both acute and chronic noncancer pain has led to significant public health and per-sonal consequences of abuse, misuse, and diversion and their resultant morbidity and mortality.[3]

Over the past 15 years significant advances have been made in our understanding of the neurobiological aspects of pain. These advances have led to a shift to mechanism-specific pain prevention and treatment approaches whenever possible. With this latter approach, the neurobiological abnormalities creating pain are identified and targeted with specific analgesics or interventions. This approach to the manage-ment of pain in the ED allows more refined and judicious use of opioid analgesics.[4] The purpose of this article is to review recent advances in the management of acute and chronic pain in the ED as well as to discuss several newer strategies and controversies.

Acute Pain

Acute pain management in the ED requires prompt recognition and assessment of a painful condition, timely initiation of safe and effective analgesia, and frequent reas-sessment and adjustment in therapy. In light of advances in the understanding of pain science, the pharmacologic armamentarium for ED analgesia has expanded dramatically over the past decade. It is recognized that most acute pain, like postop-erative pain, tends to resolve rapidly over several days; most EPs prescribe for only a few days of outpatient analgesia.[5] Similarly, there are concerns that when opioids are used too broadly for pain, the risk of long-term use, misuse, and abuse increases to unacceptable levels.[6]

Opioids

Opioids are traditionally accepted as a cornerstone in acute pain management in the ED. Their effects occur primarily through μ-opioid receptor-mediated blockade of neurotransmitter release and pain transmission. The most commonly used opioids in the ED are pure μ-receptor agonists, such as morphine, hydromorphone, or hydro-codone. Because of highly variable interindividual dose-response relationships, for pure μ-opioid agonists, dosages should be titrated upward on a case-by-case basis until satisfactory pain relief is achieved or adverse effects become unacceptable.[7,8] Several controversies surround opioid administration in the ED for acute pain, including optimal opioid selection based on the indication (clinical circumstances and context), patient variables, pain severity, optimal dose and dosing regimen, and, in particular, appropriate prescribing practices on discharge.

Parenteral (intravenous) dosing

Proponents of weight-based dosing regimens advocate for morphine dosing of 0.1 mg/kg, hydromorphone of 0.015 mg/kg, or fentanyl of 1.5 mcg/kg. However, morphine given at 0.1 mg/kg as an initial dose demonstrates inadequate pain relief in a large pro-portion of patients with acute traumatic and nontraumatic pain. Studies demonstrated less than 50% reduction in pain score (less than 3 points on the numeric rating scale [NRS]) in 67% and 47% of patients at 30 minutes and 60 minutes, respectively[9,10]; fentanyl rescue in 49% of patients with renal colic at 30 minutes[11]; and lack of efficacy at 30 minutes compared with placebo in children with abdominal pain.[12] Supporters of a fixed dosing regimen recommend administration of 4 mg of morphine or 1 mg of hydromorphone, as this regimen provided greater than 3 points change in pain score (NRS) regardless of patients' weight.[13–15] Unfortunately, fixed dosing regimens do not take into account the fact that different patients require different doses of opioids to treat similar painful conditions and that this variability in opioid dosing requirements cannot be reliably predicted. Therefore, the key to successful parenteral opioid analgesia is the titration of these analgesics. Morphine and hydromorphone titration protocols produced acceptable pain relief in 99% of and 96% of patients at 60 minutes.[16,17]

Nebulized/intranasal analgesia

Nebulized and intranasal routes of opioid administration provide rapid and reliable noninvasive analgesia in the absence of exigent intravenous (IV) access. Fentanyl is considered safe and effective when administered via nebulization at doses of 3 to 4 μg/kg and intranasally at doses 1 to 2 μg/kg to adult and pediatric patients with acute abdominal pain and acute traumatic pain.[18–20] One concern with the nebulized regimen is the potential variability in the dose actually administered, which may lead either to undertreatment of pain or to overdose. **Table 1** summarizes the dosing and titration intervals of commonly used opioids in the ED.

Patient-controlled analgesia

Patient-controlled analgesia (PCA) using morphine, hydromorphone, or fentanyl provides similar analgesic efficacy as does titrated IV analgesic and carries greater patient and nurses satisfaction.[21,22] On the other hand, the use of PCA might result in oversedation and programming errors may lead to respiratory depression and greater time, effort, and expense.[23] The overall incidence of respiratory depression in patients using PCA ranges from 0.1% to 0.8%, although higher rates of 1.1% to 3.9% have been found with concurrent basal infusion. From a risk-benefits perspective, elderly patients, patients with obstructive sleep apnea, and patients with concurrent sedatives and break-through opioid use are at greatest risk for respiratory depression and, therefore, should not be candidates for ED PCA.[23]

Table 1
Opioid dosing in the adult ED for severe acute pain

Opioids	Routes	Dosing	Pitfalls
Morphine	IV: weight based	0.1–0.15 mg/kg	Titration at 20 min: if 10-mg dose use as a drip over 5–10 min
	IV: fixed	2–4 mg	Titration at 10–15 min
	SQ	2–4 mg	Titration at 10–15 min
	IM	2–4 mg	Unpredictable response/duration of analgesia
Hydromorphone	IV: weight based	0.015 mg/kg	Titration at 10–15 min
	IV: fixed	0.25–1 mg	Titration at 10–15 min
	IM	0.25–2 mg	Unpredictable response/duration of analgesia
Fentanyl	IV: weight based	1.0–1.5 μg/kg	Titration at 10 min (if 100-μg dose, use a drip over 5–10 min)
	IV: fixed	25–50 μg	Titration at 10 min
	Nebulized	2–4 μg/kg	Use breath-actuated nebulizers (enclosed canister)
	Intranasal	1–2 μg/kg	No more than 1 mL per nostril, titration at 10–15 min

Abbreviations: IM, intramuscular; SQ, subcutaneous.

Nonsteroidal Antiinflammatory Drugs

Nonsteroidal antiinflammatory drugs (NSAIDs) have been used extensively for several decades for the management of a variety of acute and chronic painful conditions and remain among the most frequently used analgesics in the ED. They act primarily by inhibiting (reversibly) the activity of both cyclooxygenase (COX)-1 (constitutive) and COX-2 (inducible) enzymes and block the synthesis of prostaglandins and thromboxanes. NSAIDs are available in oral, rectal, topical (dermal cream), and parenteral formulations.[24,25] From a clinical perspective, their utility in the ED is limited by an analgesic ceiling (ie, nontitratable dosing) and a potentially concerning side effect profile.[26]

The analgesic ceiling refers to the dose of a drug beyond which any further dose increase will not result in additional analgesic efficacy. Thus, the analgesics ceiling for ibuprofen is 400 mg per dose (1200 mg/24 h) and for ketorolac is 10 mg per dose (10 mg/24 h).[27,28] These doses are less than those often prescribed for control of inflammation and fever. When it comes to equipotent doses of different NSAIDs, there is no difference in analgesic efficacy. For example, there is similar analgesic efficacy between oral ibuprofen at 800 mg and intramuscular (IM) ketorolac at 60 mg.[27,28] IV ketorolac is the most commonly administered parenteral NSAID in the ED; it is typically dosed at 30 mg IV and 60 mg IM, which is 3 to 6 times higher than its analgesic dose. In addition, IV ketorolac is useful in supplementing opioid and nonopioid analgesics in treating severe pain in the ED.[29] Absolute contraindications to NSAIDs use in the ED include allergy to the specific NSAID or to another in the class, active peptic ulcer disease, and tenuous renal function. Relative contraindications include prior history of gastrointestinal hemorrhage, severe hypertension, hyperkalemia, hepatic insufficiency, bleeding disorder, prior myocardial infarctions (COX-2) or stroke (COX-1), congestive heart failure, recent major vascular and cardiac surgery, pregnant patients, and elderly patients. In the ED, the most common indications for the use of an NSAIDs are renal colic, headache for which bleeding is not a likely consideration, dental pain, and musculoskeletal pain and injury. These analgesics should be used at the lowest possible dose for the shortest period of time (no more than 5 days).[24]

Acetaminophen

Acetaminophen (APAP) (paracetamol) is a p-aminophenol derivative with weak inhibitory activity of COX (COX-1, COX -2, and COX-3 isoenzymes) that translates into modest antiinflammatory and analgesic effects. APAP is available in oral, rectal, and IV formulation.[30] Earlier data in surgical and anesthesia literature advocated heavily for use of IV APAP as a part of multimodal postoperative analgesia with an ability to reduce opioid consumption by 33% to 78%.[31] Most recent trials of IV APAP, however, demonstrated a much lower opioid-sparing effect (18%–20%) and an inability to decrease opioid-induced nausea and vomiting (OINV).[32]

Several randomized controlled trials in the ED evaluated analgesic efficacy and safety of IV APAP in treating patients with renal colic, traumatic musculoskeletal pain, and migraine headache. Out of 4 renal colic trials, the use of IV APAP demonstrated similar analgesic efficacy to 0.1 mg/kg morphine in 2 trials, although the other trials demonstrated less and greater pain relief than morphine, respectively. However, all trials showed significantly less side effects in the IV APAP group (primarily nausea and vomiting) in comparison with morphine.[11,33–35] IV APAP had similar analgesic efficacy in controlling acute traumatic pain and acute migraine headache as morphine and NSAIDs with less side effects.[36,37] The greatest limitation to the use of IV APAP is the nearly 100-fold cost differential compared with oral formulations, which is likely not justified by any marginal improvement in pain relief. Perhaps when the price is lower, the cost-benefit relationship can be reassessed.

Ketamine

Ketamine is a noncompetitive N-methyl-D-aspartate (NMDA) and glutamate receptor antagonist that possesses analgesic, antihyperalgesic (opioid induced), and amnestic properties.[38] Ketamine, at subdissociative doses (also known as low-dose ketamine or analgesic dose ketamine) of 0.1 to 0.4 mg/kg, provided effective analgesia as a single agent or as an adjunct to opioids (reducing the need for opioids) in the treatment of acute traumatic and nontraumatic pain in the ED. This effective analgesia, however, must be balanced against high rates of minor adverse side effects (14%–80%), though typically short-lived and not requiring intervention.[39–41]

In addition, subdissociative dose ketamine (0.3 mg/kg IV) provided better pain relief at 5 to 15 minutes and comparable analgesic efficacy at 20 and 30 minutes in comparison with IV morphine (0.1 mg/kg) in patients with acute abdominal, flank, and back pain. However, there were higher rates of minor side effects at 5 and 15 minutes.[42,43] Subsequent case series using short infusions of low-dose ketamine (0.3 mg/kg over 10 minutes) demonstrated significantly less side effects (6%) with effective analgesia (87%) compared with bolus dosing.[44]

Furthermore, intranasal (IN) subdissociative dose ketamine administered at 1 mg/kg to children with acute traumatic limb injury demonstrates 60% decrease in pain scores at 30 minutes.[45] Similarly, 1 mg/kg IN ketamine demonstrated similar analgesic efficacy when compared with IN fentanyl (1.5 mcg/kg) at 30 minutes, though with significantly higher rates of minor side effects.[46] Lastly, IN ketamine at 0.5 to 0.75 mg/kg for patients with acute musculoskeletal trauma demonstrated significant pain relief in 88% of patients at 30 minutes with dizziness and feelings of unreality being the most frequent side effects (53% and 35%).[47]

In summary, the use of IV subdissociative dose ketamine, either alone or in combination with opioids, is safe and effective for the treatment of acute pain and may be opioid sparing. Its use has been associated with relatively high rates of minor though short-lived adverse side effects that might be reduced by using a short infusion.[44]

Local Anesthetics

Local anesthetics are widely used in the ED for topical, local, regional, intra-articular, and systemic anesthesia and analgesia. Local anesthetics (esters and amides) possess analgesic and antihyperalgesic properties by noncompetitively blocking neuronal sodium channels.[48]

Topical

Topical analgesics containing lidocaine come in patches, ointments, and creams. These formulations have been used to treat pain from acute sprains, strains, and contusions as well as variety of acute inflammatory and chronic neuropathic conditions, including postherpetic neuralgia (PHN), complex regional pain syndromes (CRPS) and painful diabetic neuropathy (PDN).[49] For example, a lidocaine patch 5% provided significant reduction of pain at rest and with movement in patients with acute herpes zoster infection with minimal side effects.[50]

Regional (ultrasound-guided nerve blocks)

Ultrasound-guided regional anesthesia (UGRA) provides substantial pain relief, reduces systemic opioid requirements, results in high degrees of patient satisfaction, and decreases resources utilization. It may replace procedural sedation for certain indications.

Studies (case series and randomized trials) evaluating UGRA (eg, interscalene, supraclavicular, and forearm blocks) with either 1% lidocaine or 0.25% bupivacaine for patients with upper extremity trauma (fractures, dislocations) or infections (abscess) demonstrated complete pain control, total muscle relaxation, and successful completion of procedures.[51–53] Similarly, studies describing UGRA for patients with lower extremity fractures or dislocations (eg, femoral nerve block, fascia iliaca compartment block) demonstrated significant pain control, decreased need for rescue analgesia, and first-attempt procedural success.[54–56] In addition, UGRA demonstrated few procedural complications, minimal need for rescue analgesia, and great patient satisfaction.[56]

Intra-articular

Intra-articular lidocaine (IAL) injection (with and without ultrasound guidance) for patients with acute shoulder dislocations has gained popularity among EPs. The available data demonstrate that IAL in the ED was associated with decreased length of stay (LOS), decreased overall cost of treatment, decreased complications rate, and modest effects on periprocedural pain relief and reduction success compared with standard reduction techniques.[57,58]

Systemic (intravenous)

Analgesic efficacy and safety of IV lidocaine has been evaluated in patients with renal colic and acute lower back pain. IV lidocaine 2% without preservatives (ie, cardiac formulation) given at 1.5 mg/kg resulted in complete resolution of renal colic pain in 87% of patients in case series and significant pain decrease (greater than 3 on NRS) in 90% of subjects in randomized controlled trials. The most common (transient) side effects were dizziness and nausea.[59,60] In addition, administration of 100 mg IV lidocaine improved the pain score in patients with acute lower back pain at 60 minutes but required rescue analgesia in 65% of patients.[61] Although promising, this therapy will need to be studied in larger populations with underlying cardiac disease before it can be broadly used.

Nitrous Oxide

Nitrous oxide is a colorless, tasteless gas that provides analgesia by stabilizing the neurons in the brain to prevent action potential propagation and by interacting with the endogenous opioid system via a partial agonism at μ and κ opioid receptors.[62] Nitrous oxide mixture (50:50) provided significant analgesia and reduction in anxiety to 1201 patients in a rural emergency services system, with 21% of patients developing minor side effects, mostly dizziness or lightheadedness.[63] Nitrous oxide in combination with hematoma block was found to be more effective than ketamine/midazolam combination in relieving pain, to have shorter recovery times, and fewer adverse side effects for patients with forearm fracture.[64] Nitrous oxide (50:50 mixture) demonstrated similar analgesic efficacy to IV fentanyl (2 μg/kg) and no difference in adverse effects in patients with long bone fracture.[65]

Channels/enzymes/receptors Targeted Analgesia Concept

The channels/enzymes/receptors targeted analgesia (CERTA) concept is based on our improved understanding of the neurobiological aspect of pain with a shift from a symptom-based approach to pain to a mechanistic approach. This targeted analgesic approach allows for a broader utilization of synergistic combinations of nonopioid analgesia and more refined and judicious (rescue) use of opioids.[4] These synergistic combinations result in greater analgesia, fewer side effects, lesser sedation, and shorter LOS. An example of this concept would include a combination of COX enzymes inhibitor (ketorolac) with a sodium channel-blocking agent (IV lidocaine) for patients with renal colic. Another example would include a combination of NMDA-receptor antagonist (ketamine) with sodium channel blockade (lidocaine via UGRA) for acute traumatic musculoskeletal pain. **Table 2** summarizes possible combinations and their utilizations in the ED for pain management.

CHRONIC PAIN

Chronic noncancer pain is a multifactorial entity affecting social, behavioral, and psychological aspects of peoples' lives and society in general. Chronic pain carries a significant societal burden that reportedly affects 31% of the adult population in the United States and costs between $560 and $635 billion annually, which is greater than the annual costs of heart disease ($309 billion), cancer ($243 billion), and diabetes ($188 billion).[66]

Unfortunately, as the use of opioid analgesics for treatment of chronic noncancer pain accelerated over the past 2 decades, significant increases in prescription opioid misuse, abuse, addiction, diversion, and opioid-related mortality have occurred. Between 1997 and 2007, the quantity of prescribed opioids increased by 866% overall and 380% for oxycodone and hydrocodone, respectively. Between 1997 and 2013, 175,000 deaths were reported due to prescription opioid overdose and the rates of addiction treatment from prescription opioid abuse increased by 900%.[67]

The rate of prescription opioid misuse (ie, not taking medication exactly as directed) among patients with chronic pain is as high as 24%, and rates of opioid use disorder are 26%.[68,69] Opioids may also cause hyperalgesia (heightened pain perception to a noxious stimulus), especially when taken in high doses over prolonged periods of time-.[69] Thus, the complexity of chronic pain requires a very comprehensive, multidisciplinary approach to its evaluation and management that includes identification and treatment of exacerbating factors, utilization of psychological treatment modalities, administration of nonopioid and adjuvant analgesics, treatment of associated behavioral disorders, and restoration of sleep and daily activities. Only after these measures are optimized should a trial of opioid therapy, or continuation of existing opioid therapy, be considered.[70]

The fast-paced environment of the ED, geared toward rapid treatment of acute injuries or illnesses, precludes EPs from investing significant amounts of time to communicate with patients with chronic pain, access past medical records, adequately assess patients' risk for opioid abuse and misuse, or verify patient-physician agreements.[70,71]

However, EPs can use state prescription drug monitoring programs (PDMPs) where accessible to ensure patients' safe opioid use by avoiding excessive dosing and drug interactions and by identifying aberrant use behaviors, or doctor shopping. In one study, implementation of such programs resulted in a change of the clinical management in 41% of cases, with most patients (61%) receiving less opioid analgesic than originally planned and 39% receiving more.[72] Another trial demonstrated fair agreement between emergency provider impression of drug-seeking behavior and that suggested by the PDMP ($\kappa = 0.30$), with a resultant change in prescribing opioids at discharge in 9.5% of cases.[73]

The American College of Emergency Physicians and the American Academy of Emergency Medicine have created recommendations for EPs to assist in their analgesic practices for patients with chronic noncancer pain[74,75] (**Box 1**). However, the

Table 2
CERTA concept

Target Site	Medications/Dosing	Indications	Pain Syndromes
Sodium channels blockers	*Lidocaine:* Topical: 5% Lidoderm patch	Chronic/acute MSK pain	Tendinitis, osteoarthritis, contusion Traumatic injuries
	Local: 1%–2% (4 mg/kg max) Regional: 1%–2% (4 mg/kg max)	Acute MSK pain	Traumatic injuries (fractures, dislocations)
	Intra-articular: 1% (20–30 mL)	Acute MSK pain	Dislocations (shoulder)
	Systemic IV: 2% cardiac Lidocaine (1.5–2.0 mg/kg, max 200 mg)	Acute visceral pain	Renal colic
	Bupivacaine: Local: 0.25%–0.5% (2.5 mg/kg max)	Acute MSK pain	Traumatic injuries (lacerations)
	Regional: 0.25%–0.5% (2.5 mg/kg max)	Acute MSK pain	Traumatic injuries (fractures, dislocations)
	Nortriptyline: 25 mg po	Chronic neuropathic pain	Postherpetic neuralgia, sciatica, diabetic neuropathy
	Amitriptyline: 10 mg po	—	
Calcium channels (central) blockers	Gabapentin: 100–300 mg Pregabalin: 25 mg po	Acute postoperative pain Acute neuropathic pain Chronic neuropathic pain	Nerve palsies, neuralgias Diabetic neuropathy Postherpetic Neuropathy, sciatica, fibromyalgia
Cox-1, -2, -3 enzymes inhibitors	*NSAIDs:* Ibuprofen: 400 mg po Naproxen: 250–375–500 mg po	Acute MSK pain (trauma), headache, inflammatory pain chronic MSK pain	Sprains, strains, contusions Chronic osteoarthritis, tendinopathies
	Ketorolac IV: 10–30 mg	Acute MSK pain, acute abdominal pain	Renal colic, abdominal pain (nontraumatic), back pain, headache
	Topical: Diclofenac 1% gel Diclofenac 1.3% patch	Acute MSK pain	Sprains, strains, contusions Chronic osteoarthritis, tendinopathies
NMDA/glutamate receptors antagonists	Ketamine (subdissociative dosing): IV bolus: 0.1–0.4 mg/kg over 10 min IV infusion: 0.15–0.25 mg/kg/h IN: 0.75–1.0 mg/kg SQ: 0.1–0.4 mg/kg	Acute pain, opioid-tolerant pain, chronic pain	Traumatic pain, abdominal/flank/back pain, sickle cell pain, sciatica, abdominal migraine, neuropathic pain

Drug class	Medication/dose	Indication	Use
Central alpha 1, 2 receptors agonists	Clonidine IV: 0.5–1.0 μg/kg	Acute pain, chronic pain	Adjunct to local anesthetics, opioids, ketamine for acute traumatic/nontraumatic pain
	Dexemedetomidine IV: −0.5–1.0 μg/kg bolus −0.1–0.5 μg/kg/h infusion	Acute pain, neuropathic pain, opioid-resistant pain	Sickle cell pain, CRPS, severe sciatica
Opioid receptors agonists (μ-receptors)	Morphine: (IV, SQ, remove) weight based, fixed Hydromorphone (IV, IM): weight based, fixed Fentanyl (IV, IN, nebulization): weight based, fixed	Acute traumatic/nontraumatic pain	Acute MSK pain (fractures), acute abdominal pain, acute traumatic/nontraumatic pain
GABA receptors agonist	Diprivan (propofol) IV: 10 mg q 5 min	Acute headache	Intractable migraine headache
Volatile anesthetic (endogenous opioid receptors agonist)	Nitrous oxide: 50/50 concentration 70/30 concentration	Acute pain: traumatic/nontraumatic	Fractures, dislocations, adjunct to local/regional blocks, opioids
D1-2 receptors antagonists	Haldol IV: 1–2 mg Droperidol IV: 2–5 mg Metoclopramide IV: 10–20 mg Prochlorperazine IV: 10 mg Chlorpromazine IV: 5–50 mg IV	Acute pain	Migraine headache, chronic abdominal angina
5HT-2, 5HT-3 receptors antagonists	Metoclopramide IV: 10–20 mg Haldol IV: 1–2 mg Droperidol IV: 2–5 mg	Acute pain	Migraine headache
5HT-1 agonists	Sumatriptan SQ: 4–6 mg	Acute pain	Migraine headache Cluster headache

---

Box 1

Opioid-prescribing guidelines in treatment of chronic noncancer pain in the ED

1. The physician should honor existing patient-physician pain contracts and treatment agreements and consider past prescription patterns from information sources, such as centralized or state-specific PDMPs.

2. The physicians should avoid the routine prescribing of outpatient opioids for patients with acute exacerbation of chronic noncancer pain seen in the ED.

3. The physician should address acute exacerbation of chronic noncancer pain by using nonopioid analgesics, nonpharmacologic therapies, or referral to pain clinic/specialist for arranged follow-up if patients do not have a private physician.

4. If opioids are to prescribed on discharge, the prescription should be for the lowest practical dose for a limited duration (3 days supply), and the physician should consider patients' risk for opioid misuse, abuse, or diversion.

5. The physician should avoid initiating long-acting or extended-release opioids, such as oxycodone and methadone.

6. The physician should not replace lost, stolen, or destroyed prescription and should not refill chronic opioid prescriptions including ER/LA opioids.

7. The physician should avoid prescribing opioids to patients currently taking sedative-hypnotics medications or concurrent opioid analgesics.

8. The physician must provided information to patients regarding risks of using opioid analgesics, such as overdose, dependence, and addiction, as well as educate patients about safe storage and proper medication disposal.

9. The physician should offer an alternative to opioid analgesics to patients and should actively involve patients in their analgesic decision making.

Data from Cantrill SV, Brown MD, Carlisle RJ, et al. Clinical policy: critical issues in the prescribing of opioids for adult patients in the emergency department. Ann Emerg Med 2012;60(4):499–525; and Cheng D, Majlesi N. Emergency department opioid prescribing guidelines for the treatment of non-cancer related pain. AAEM Position Statement. 2013. Available at: http://www.aaem.org/UserFiles/file/Emergency-Department-Opoid-Prescribing-Guidelines.pdf.

---

ideal path of safe and effective chronic pain management in the ED should focus on provision of education on the effectiveness and safety of all analgesics (including NSAIDs, opioids, nonopioid analgesics), evaluation of risk of opioid abuse and misuse, and on engaging patients in the decision making to use opioids. Discussion with and referral to their primary care provider or pain medicine physician should be performed if practical. Each EP must promote safe and effective patient-centered analgesia by using informed prescribing through the use of aids, such as the PDMPs and analgesic prescribing guidelines, along with an eye toward the public health risks (eg, diversion) of opioid analgesics.[69]

SUMMARY

The ED is a primary setting for medical care for many patients presenting with traumatic and nontraumatic painful conditions. In providing effective care to the populations served by the ED, EPs have a great responsibility to relieve pain by all possible appropriate means in a timely, efficient, and safe manner. The improvement in our understanding of the neurobiology of pain has lead to a great deal of utilization of nonopioid analgesia in the ED and, simultaneously, has led to more rational and safer opioid prescribing practices. We must promote patient-centered, pain-syndrome targeted analgesia in the ED through education, collaboration, and exploration of more efficient and safer analgesics practices in the ED.

REFERENCES

1. Chang HY, Daubresse M, Kruszewski SP, et al. Prevalence and treatment of pain in EDs in the United States, 2000 to 2010. Am J Emerg Med 2014;32(5):421–31.
2. Green SM. There is oligo-evidence for oligoanalgesia. Ann Emerg Med 2012;60: 212–4.
3. Warner M, Hedegaard H, Chen LH. Trends in drug-poisoning deaths involving opioid analgesics and heroin: United States, 1999–2012. NCHS Health E-Stat. Hyattsville (MD): National Centers for Health Statistics; 2014. Available at: www.cdc.gov/nchs/data/hestat/drug_poisoning/drug_poisoning_deaths_1999-2012.pdf.
4. Ducharme J. Non-opioid pain medications to consider for emergency department patients. Available at: http://www.acepnow.com/article/non-opioid-pain-medications-consider-emergency-department-patients/. Accessed February 11, 2015.
5. Rodgers J, Cunningham K, Fitzgerald K, et al. Opioid consumption following outpatient upper extremity surgery. J Hand Surg Am 2012;37(4):645–50.
6. Alam A, Gomes T, Zheng H, et al. Long-term analgesic use after low risk surgery: a retrospective cohort study. Arch Intern Med 2012;172:425–30.
7. Rowbotham DJ, Serrano-Gomez A, Heffernan A. Clinical pharmacology: opioids. In: Macintyre PE, editor. Clinical pain management (acute pain). 2nd edition. London: Hodder & Stoughton Limited; 2008. p. 68–79.
8. Patanwala AE, Keim SM, Erstad BL. Intravenous opioids for severe acute pain in the emergency department. Ann Pharmacother 2010;44(11):1800–9.
9. Bijur PE, Kenny MK, Gallagher EJ. Intravenous morphine at 0.1 mg/kg is not effective for controlling severe acute pain in the majority of patients. Ann Emerg Med 2005;46:362–7.
10. Birnbaum A, Esses D, Bijur PE, et al. Randomized double-blind placebo- controlled trial of two intravenous morphine dosages (0.10 mg/kg and 0.15 mg/kg) in emergency department patients with moderate to severe acute pain. Ann Emerg Med 2007;49(4):445–53.
11. Bektas F, Eken C, Karadeniz O, et al. Intravenous paracetamol or morphine for the treatment of renal colic: a randomized, placebo-controlled trial. Ann Emerg Med 2009;54(4):568–74.
12. Bailey B, Bergeron S, Gravel J, et al. Efficacy and impact of intravenous morphine before surgical consultation in children with right lower quadrant pain suggestive of appendicitis: a randomized controlled trial. Ann Emerg Med 2007;50:371–8.
13. Patanwala AE, Edwards CJ, Stolz L, et al. Should morphine dosing be weight based for analgesia in the emergency department? J Opioid Manag 2012; 8(1):51–5.
14. Patanwala AE, Holmes KL, Erstad BL. Analgesic response to morphine in obese and morbidly obese patients in the emergency department. Emerg Med J 2014; 31(2):139–42.
15. Xia S, Chew E, Choe D, et al. No correlation between body size and hydromorphone analgesia in obese patients in ED. Am J Emerg Med 2015;33(10):1522–3.
16. Lvovschi V, Auburn F, Bonnet P, et al. Intravenous morphine titration to treat severe pain in the ED. Am J Emerg Med 2008;26:676–82.
17. Chang AK, Bijur PE, Campbell CM, et al. Safety and efficacy of rapid titration using 1mg doses of intravenous hydromorphone in emergency department

patients with acute severe pain: the "1+1" protocol. Ann Emerg Med 2009;54(2): 221–5.

18. Miner JR, Kletti C, Herold M, et al. Randomized clinical trial of nebulized fentanyl citrate versus i.v. fentanyl citrate in children presenting to the emergency department with acute pain. Acad Emerg Med 2007;14:895–8.

19. Furyk JS, Grabowski WJ, Black LH. Nebulized fentanyl versus intravenous morphine in children with suspected limb fractures in the emergency department: a randomized controlled trial. Emerg Med Australas 2009;21:203–9.

20. Borland M, Jacobs I, King B, et al. A randomized controlled trial comparing intranasal fentanyl to intravenous morphine for managing acute pain in children in the emergency department. Ann Emerg Med 2007;49:335–40.

21. Evans E, Turley N, Robinson N, et al. Randomised controlled trial of patient controlled analgesia compared with nurse delivered analgesia in an emergency department. Emerg Med J 2005;22:25–9.

22. Rahman NH, DeSilva T. A randomized controlled trial of patient-controlled analgesia compared with boluses of analgesia for the control of acute traumatic pain in the emergency department. J Emerg Med 2012;43(6):951–7.

23. Macintyre PE. Safety and efficacy of patient-controlled analgesia. Br J Anaesth 2001;87(1):36–46.

24. Jones SF, O'Donnell AM. Clinical Pharmacology: traditional NSAIDs and selective COX-2 inhibitors. In: Macintyre PE, Walker SM, Rowbotham DJ, et al, editors. Clinical pain management (acute pain). 2nd edition. London: Hodder & Stoughton Limited; 2008. p. 68–79.

25. Thomas SH. Management of pain in the emergency department. ISRN Emerg Med 2013;2013. Available at: http://www.hindawi.com/journals/isrn/2013/583132/.

26. Castellsague J, Riera-Guardia N, Calingaert B, et al. Individual NSAIDs and upper gastrointestinal complications: a systematic review and meta-analysis of observational studies (the SOS project). Drug Saf 2012;35:1127–46.

27. Wright JM, Price SD, Watson WA. NSAID use and efficacy in the emergency department: single doses of oral ibuprofen versus intramuscular ketorolac. Ann Pharmacother 1994;28(3):309–12.

28. Turturro MA, Paris PM, Seaberg DC. Intramuscular ketorolac versus oral ibuprofen in acute musculoskeletal pain. Ann Emerg Med 1995;26(2):117–20.

29. Catapano MS. The analgesic efficacy of ketorolac for acute pain [review]. J Emerg Med 1996;14(1):67–75.

30. Wiffen P. Clinical Pharmacology: paracetamol and compund analgesics. In: Macintyre PE, Walker SM, Rowbotham DJ, et al, editors. Clinical pain management (acute pain). 2nd edition. London: Hodder & Stoughton Limited; 2008. p. 84–93.

31. Viscusi ER, Singla N, Gonzalez A, et al. IV acetaminophen improves pain management and reduces opioid requirements in surgical patients. Available at: http://www.anesthesiologynews.com/download/SR122_WM.pdf. Accessed February 6, 2016.

32. Yeh YC, Reddy P. Clinical and economic evidence for intravenous acetaminophen. Pharmacotherapy 2012;32(6):559–79.

33. Serinken M, Eken C, Turkcuer I, et al. Intravenous paracetamol versus morphine for renal colic in the emergency department: a randomised double-blind controlled trial. Emerg Med J 2012;29(11):902–5.

34. Azizkhani R, Pourafzali SM, Baloochestani E, et al. Comparing the analgesic effect of intravenous acetaminophen and morphine on patients with renal colic pain referring to the emergency department: A randomized controlled trial. J Res Med Sci 2013;18(9):772–6.

35. Masoumi K, Forouzan A, Asgari Darian A, et al. Comparison of clinical efficacy of intravenous acetaminophen with intravenous morphine in acute renal colic: a randomized, double-blind, controlled trial. Emerg Med Int 2014;2014:571326.
36. Craig M, Jeavons R, Probert J, et al. Randomised comparison of intravenous paracetamol and intravenous morphine for acute traumatic limb pain in the emergency department. Emerg Med J 2012;29(1):37–9.
37. Turkcuer I, Serinken M, Eken C, et al. Intravenous paracetamol versus dexketoprofen in acute migraine attack in the emergency department: a randomised clinical trial. Emerg Med J 2014;31(3):182–5.
38. Kurdi MS, Theerth KA, Deva RS. Ketamine: Current applications in anesthesia, pain, and critical care. Anesth Essays Res 2014;8(3):283–9.
39. Galinski M, Dolveck F, Combes X, et al. Management of severe acute pain in emergency settings: ketamine reduces morphine consumption. Am J Emerg Med 2007;25(4):385–90.
40. Ahern TL, Herring AA, Stone MB, et al. Effective analgesia with low-dose ketamine and reduced dose hydromorphone in ED patients with severe pain. Am J Emerg Med 2013;31(5):847–51.
41. Beaudoin FL, Lin C, Guan W, et al. Low-dose ketamine improves pain relief in patients receiving intravenous opioids for acute pain in the emergency department: results of a randomized, double-blind, clinical trial. Acad Emerg Med 2014;21(11):1193–202.
42. Miller JP, Schauer SG, Ganem VJ, et al. Low-dose ketamine vs morphine for acute pain in the ED: a randomized controlled trial. Am J Emerg Med 2015;33(3):402–8.
43. Motov S, Rockoff B, Cohen V, et al. Intravenous subdissociative-dose ketamine versus morphine for analgesia in the emergency department: a randomized controlled trial. Ann Emerg Med 2015;66(3):222–9.e1.
44. Goltser A, Soleyman-Zomalan E, Kresch F, et al. Short (low-dose) ketamine infusion for managing acute pain in the ED: case-report series. Am J Emerg Med 2015;33(4):601.e5–7.
45. Yeaman F, Oakley E, Meek R, et al. Sub-dissociative dose intranasal ketamine for limb injury pain in children in the emergency department:a pilot study. Emerg Med Australas 2013;25(2):161–7.
46. Graudins A, Meek R, Egerton-Warburton D, et al. The PICHFORK (Pain in Children Fentanyl or Ketamine) trial: a randomized controlled trial comparing intranasal ketamine and fentanyl for the relief of moderate to severe pain in children with limb injuries. Ann Emerg Med 2015;65(3):248–54.
47. Andolfatto G, Willman E, Joo D, et al. Intranasal ketamine for analgesia in the emergency department: a prospective observational series. Acad Emerg Med 2013;20(10):1050–4.
48. McGhie J, Serpell MG. Clinical pharmacology: local anesthetics. In: Macintyre PE, Walker SM, Rowbotham DJ, et al, editors. Clinical pain management (acute pain). 2nd edition. London: Hodder & Stoughton Limited; 2008. p. 113–29.
49. D'Arcy Y. Targeted topical analgesics for acute pain. Pain Med News 2014;12(12): 56–63. Available at: http://www.painmedicinenews.com/Review-Articles/Article/12-14/Targeted-Topical-Analgesics-For-Acute-Pain/28992. Accessed February 6, 2016.
50. Lin PL, Fan SZ, Huang CH, et al. Analgesic effect of lidocaine patch 5% in the treatment of acute herpes zoster: a double-blind and vehicle-controlled study. Reg Anesth Pain Med 2008;33(4):320–5.
51. Blaivas M, Lyon M. Ultrasound-guided interscalene block for shoulder dislocation reduction in the ED. Am J Emerg Med 2006;24(3):293–6.

52. Stone MB, Price DD, Wang R. Ultrasound-guided supraclavicular block for the treatment of upper extremity fractures, dislocations, and abscesses in the ED. Am J Emerg Med 2007;25(4):472–5.

53. Liebmann O, Price D, Mills C, et al. Feasibility of forearm ultrasonography-guided nerve blocks of the radial, ulnar, and median nerves for hand procedures in the emergency department. Ann Emerg Med 2006;48(5):558–62.

54. Haines L, Dickman E, Ayvazyan S, et al. Ultrasound-guided fascia iliaca compartment block for hip fractures in the emergency department. J Emerg Med 2012; 43(4):692–7.

55. Beaudoin FL, Nagdev A, Merchant RC, et al. Ultrasound-guided femoral nerve blocks in elderly patients with hip fractures. Am J Emerg Med 2010;28(1):76–81.

56. Bhoi S, Sinha TP, Rodha M, et al. Feasibility and safety of ultrasound-guided nerve block for management of limb injuries by emergency care physicians. J Emerg Trauma Shock 2012;5(1):28–32.

57. Fitch RW, Kuhn JE. Intraarticular lidocaine versus intravenous procedural sedation with narcotics and benzodiazepines for reduction of the dislocated shoulder: a systematic review. Acad Emerg Med 2008;15(8):703–8.

58. Wakai A, O'Sullivan R, McCabe A. Intra-articular lignocaine versus intravenous analgesia with or without sedation for manual reduction of acute anterior shoulder dislocation in adults. Cochrane Database Syst Rev 2011;(4):CD004919.

59. Soleimanpour H, Hassanzadeh K, Mohammadi DA, et al. Parenteral lidocaine for treatment of intractable renal colic: a case series. J Med Case Rep 2011;5:256.

60. Soleimanpour H, Hassanzadeh K, Vaezi H, et al. Effectiveness of intravenous lidocaine versus intravenous morphine for patients with renal colic in the emergency department. BMC Urol 2012;12:13.

61. Tanen DA, Shimada M, Danish DC, et al. Intravenous lidocaine for the emergency department treatment of acute radicular low back pain, a randomized controlled trial. J Emerg Med 2014;47(1):119–24.

62. Tziavrangos E, Schug SA. Clinical pharmacology: other adjuvants. In: Macintyre PE, Walker SM, Rowbotham DJ, et al, editors. Clinical pain management (acute pain). 2nd edition. London: Hodder & Stoughton Limited; 2008. p. 97–8.

63. Johnson JC, Atherton GL. Effectiveness of nitrous oxide in a rural EMS system. J Emerg Med 1991;9(1–2):45–53.

64. Luhmann JD, Schootman M, Luhmann SJ, et al. A randomized comparison of nitrous oxide plus hematoma block versus ketamine plus midazolam for emergency department forearm fracture reduction in children. Pediatrics 2006; 118(4):e1078–86.

65. Kariman H, Majidi A, Amini A, et al. Nitrous oxide/oxygen compared with fentanyl in reducing pain among adults with isolated extremity trauma: a randomized trial. Emerg Med Australas 2011;23(6):761–8.

66. Gaskin DJ, Richard P. The economic costs of pain in the United States. In: relieving pain in America: a blueprint for transforming prevention, care, education, and research. 2011. Available at: http://www.ncbi.nlm.nih.gov/books/NBK91497/pdf/Bookshelf_NBK91497.pdf. Accessed February 6, 2016.

67. Manchikanti L, Helm S 2nd, Fellows B, et al. Opioid epidemic in the United States. Pain Physician 2012;15(3 Suppl):ES9–38.

68. Hoppe JA, Houghland J, Yaron M, et al. Prescription history of emergency department patients prescribed opioids. West J Emerg Med 2013;14(3):247–52.

69. Perrone J, Nelson LS, Yealy DM. Choosing analgesics wisely: what we know (and still need to know) about long-term consequences of opioids. Ann Emerg Med 2015;65(5):500–2.

70. Berland D, Rodgers P. Rational use of opioids for management of chronic non-terminal pain. Am Fam Physician 2012;86(3):252–8.
71. Gauntlett-Gilbert J, Rodham K, Jordan A, et al. Emergency department staff attitudes toward people presenting in chronic pain: a qualitative study. Pain Med 2015;16(11):2065–74.
72. Baehren DF, Marco CA, Droz DE, et al. A statewide prescription monitoring program affects emergency department prescribing behaviors. Ann Emerg Med 2010;56(1):19–23.e1-3.
73. Weiner SG, Griggs CA, Mitchell PM, et al. Clinician impression versus prescription drug monitoring program criteria in the assessment of drug-seeking behavior in the emergency department. Ann Emerg Med 2013;62(4):281–9.
74. Cantrill SV, Brown MD, Carlisle RJ, et al. Clinical policy: critical issues in the prescribing of opioids for adult patients in the emergency department. Ann Emerg Med 2012;60(4):499–525.
75. Cheng D, Majlesi N. Emergency department opioid prescribing guidelines for the treatment of non-cancer related pain. Milwaukee (WI): AAEM Position Statement; 2013. Available at: http://www.aaem.org/UserFiles/file/Emergency-Department-Opoid-Prescribing-Guidelines.pdf.

Managing Opioid-Tolerant Patients in the Perioperative Surgical Home

John T. Wenzel, MD*, Eric S. Schwenk, MD,
Jaime L. Baratta, MD, Eugene R. Viscusi, MD

KEYWORDS

- Opioid tolerance • Multimodal analgesia • Perioperative surgical home
- Buprenorphine

KEY POINTS

- In the perioperative surgical home model, anesthesiologists are well positioned to manage complex patients, including those who are opioid-tolerant, because of their training and expertise in pharmacology.
- Opioid-tolerant patients present challenges for postoperative analgesia, posing dual risks of poor pain control and medication-related toxicity.
- Reduction of opioids through regional anesthesia techniques and multimodal nonopioid agents can improve analgesia and minimize opioid-related complications in the high-risk opioid-tolerant population.

INTRODUCTION

Acute pain is a major concern of many patients preparing to undergo surgery. The incidence of postoperative acute pain varies widely in the literature. It has been reported as high as 80% and is likely underreported.[1] Such data suggest that uncontrolled acute postoperative pain continues to be an unmet need and a target for improvement. This is further compounded in opioid-tolerant patients receiving chronic opioids at baseline. While preparing to manage opioid-tolerant patients, mechanisms underlying chronic postsurgical pain (CPSP), acute opioid tolerance, and opioid-induced hyperalgesia (OIH) are poorly understood but highly relevant. The emerging model of the perioperative surgical home (PSH) puts anesthesiologists in position to best

Disclosures: J.T. Wenzel, E.S. Schwenk and J.L. Baratta have no financial disclosures. E.R. Viscusi: research grants to author's institution, AcelRx, Cumberland, and Pacira; consulting/honoraria, AcelRx, Malinckrodt, The Medicines Company, Merck, Salix, Pacira, and Trevena.
Department of Anesthesiology, Sidney Kimmel Medical College, Thomas Jefferson University, Suite 8130, Gibbon Building, 111 South 11th Street, Philadelphia, PA 19107, USA
* Corresponding author.
E-mail address: John.Wenzel@jefferson.edu

Anesthesiology Clin 34 (2016) 287–301
http://dx.doi.org/10.1016/j.anclin.2016.01.005
1932-2275/16/$ – see front matter © 2016 Elsevier Inc. All rights reserved.

address complicated patients, particularly those with preexisting chronic pain conditions and who are opioid tolerant as a result of chronic opioid therapy.

The Perioperative Surgical Home

The PSH has been supported by the American Society of Anesthesiologists (ASA) to improve outcomes while improving efficiency, broadening the role of the anesthesiologist in preoperative, intraoperative, and postoperative care. It is defined by the ASA as "a patient-centered and physician-led multidisciplinary and team-based system of coordinated care that guides the patient throughout the entire surgical experience."[2] The Triple Aim goals of the PSH as described by Berwick and colleagues[3] include

1. Improving the individual experience of care
2. Improving the health of populations
3. Reducing the per capita cost of care

The PSH for surgical patients has been compared with the patient-centered medical home (PCMH) for primary care. Recent data suggest that the PCMH improves outcomes and reduces costs.[4] Development of the PSH requires the support of hospital administration and collaboration of surgeons and anesthesiologists. Anesthesiologists are particularly well suited to staff the PSH[4] as the physician team leader. Because many institutions do not have an existing preoperative anesthesia clinic, development of a PSH can be financially challenging. If there is institutional support or desire for PSH development, the institution and anesthesia practice need to be financially aligned with an agreement to support funding.[4] Compensation for staffing also needs to be considered. Hospital administration may be willing to compensate anesthesiologists for this practice if a financial benefit can be demonstrated. Reimbursement for anesthesiologists may mirror that of internists in the PCMH, as the Centers for Medicare and Medicaid Services have recognized the value of the PCMH.[2] Future payment models that include bundled payments for services may make anesthesiologist compensation complicated.

Once the PSH is implemented, services begin with early patient engagement after the decision for surgery is made. The surgical experience is treated as a fluid continuum rather than discrete presurgical, intrasurgical, and postsurgical phases. It involves appropriate risk stratification and preoperative testing, decreased redundancy in testing, improved operating room efficiency, decreased variability through the use of evidence-based surgical care pathways, and postsurgical care initiatives.[5] The authors focus on management of opioid-tolerant patients within the PSH.

Opioids

Opioids remain a mainstay of analgesia regimens for surgical patients. Prescriptions for opioids as well as the increased incidence of prescription opioid abuse have been increasing in recent years, especially in the United States and Canada.[6] Opioid-related deaths and adverse events have seen a similar spike.[6] Yet, despite the increased use of opioid medications to manage pain and improve function, there remains a serious and significant mismatch between the number of prescriptions issued and positive end outcomes of pain care in the United States.[7] In some patients, chronic opioid exposure, especially at high doses, has been attributed to a progressive reduction in analgesia while increasing risks of opioid tolerance, opioid-induced hyperalgesia, and medication misuse.[8] These issues come into focus when patients on chronic opioid therapy have indications for surgery.

Opioid Tolerance

- It is a phenomenon whereby increasing opioid doses are required for analgesia because of a desensitization of pain signaling at the opioid receptor.[9]
- Acute opioid tolerance may develop rapidly in patients who are opioid-naïve.[10]
- Patients exposed to high intraoperative opioid doses have demonstrated increased postoperative pain and opioid requirements.
- These higher opioid doses are associated with an increased risk of adverse events.[9]

Opioid-Induced Hyperalgesia

- OIH is nociceptive sensitization likely caused by neuroplastic changes in the central and peripheral nervous systems caused by opioid exposure, leading to paradoxic worsening of pain with increasing opioid doses.
- Remifentanil has been particularly implicated; but it may occur with acute or chronic exposure, high or low doses, and any opioid or route of administration.[11]
- Prevalence of OIH is likely underappreciated as its diagnosis can be very challenging and it can be confused with tolerance, worsening disease, or even opioid withdrawal.
- When OIH is suspected, opioid dose reduction may improve analgesia. Other proposed treatments include opioid rotation, N-methyl-D-aspartate (NMDA) receptor antagonists (ketamine, memantine, dextromethorphan), interventional pain management, or behavioral management.[11]
- Rotation to methadone is of particular interest because it is both a mu-receptor opioid agonist and an NMDA-receptor antagonist.

Managing acute postoperative pain may be especially challenging in opioid-tolerant patients; increasing doses of opioids to overcome tolerance is a poor management strategy, as this may result in unwanted opioid side effects, including sedation, respiratory depression, ileus, and paradoxic worsening of pain. Multimodal analgesia involves the incorporation of several medications with unique mechanisms of action in an effort to improve analgesia and minimize the side effects of any one class of medication, especially opioids. These patients may benefit the most from preoperative optimization of their pain regimen, context-appropriate selection of intraoperative anesthetic techniques, and a multimodal postoperative analgesic plan.

PREOPERATIVE ASSESSMENT

In the PSH, the preoperative assessment begins in the preoperative clinic rather than at the bedside on the day of surgery. Patients often encounter their anesthesiologist for the first time in the presurgery holding area minutes before surgery, whereas a previously scheduled comprehensive assessment in the clinic affords time to enact a management plan for opioid-tolerant patients. This anticipatory planning and care coordination also creates the opportunity to provide perioperative education, to set expectations, and alleviate patient anxiety. Managing patient expectations for pain management is critical to success and enhances patient satisfaction. Both surgeon and anesthesiologist should be attuned to early identification and management of opioid-tolerant patients.

Assessment begins with a thorough history and physical examination and includes elucidation of the location and nature of chronic pain as well as the degree of functional impairment. Particular attention should be paid to patients' current pain regimen, including exact doses, schedule, routes of administration, prescriber, and effects (positive and negative). A complete history includes past medication use and experiences (**Box 1**). Patients who cannot provide evidence of accountability for their

---

Box 1
Components of the preoperative assessment for opioid-tolerant patients

- Clarification of preexisting pain and functional limitations
- Current opioid medications, including dose, frequency, and any changes in dose in the past 6 months
- Current opioid prescriber and dispensing pharmacy
- Current nonopioid analgesics (eg, acetaminophen, nonsteroidal antiinflammatory drugs, cyclooxygenase-2 inhibitors, antineuropathic agents, benzodiazepines, muscle relaxants)
- Past opioid medications and their effectiveness and tolerability of side effect profile
- Review of potential misuse or abuse of opioids
- Discussion of expectations and anticipated level of pain associated with the particular procedure (mild, moderate, severe), including perceptions from past surgical experiences

---

opioids justify additional exploration into opioid abuse, misuse, or diversion. A urine drug screen may be useful to determine potential substance misuse, abuse, or diversion. In the face of active, undiagnosed substance abuse, a joint decision between the surgeon and anesthesiologist should be made, weighing the risks of the abuse on both the patients' current health and surgical outcome. A more detailed discussion of substance abuse is out of the scope of this article.

The nature of the proposed surgery is important in determining the anesthetic and analgesic plan. Is it major surgery requiring hospital admission with high levels of anticipated pain? On the other hand, is discharge home on the same day anticipated? Is the procedure and medical circumstances of patients suitable for a regional anesthetic technique? Would any drugs or techniques be contraindicated because of patient characteristics (eg, renal or liver disease) or surgical type (eg, positioning, bleeding risk, or bone healing)?

Taking into account patients' medical history, planned surgery, current therapies, and existing and anticipated pain, the anesthesiologist may tailor a specific anesthetic plan that involves a combination of preemptive analgesia, regional techniques, intraoperative agents, and postoperative multimodal analgesia. Multimodal regimens are especially important for opioid-tolerant patients, with the goals of adequate analgesia, prevention of CPSP, and minimization of opioids and their associated adverse events. Chronic exposure to opioids reduces drug efficacy, requiring increasing doses to achieve similar analgesic effects. These patients may be at an increased risk when compared with opioid-naïve patients, whereby increasing dosages to improve efficacy increases the risk of adverse events, most significantly respiratory depression. Additionally, opioid-tolerant patients presenting for surgery may have altered pain sensitivity that includes generalized hyperalgesia or ill-defined pain remote to the surgical site.[12] We are, therefore, left to maximize the utility of nonopioid agents and regional techniques.

The advantages of a patient-specific analgesic plan are several-fold: first, patients will be well informed about expectations and will not be expected to make decisions about their care immediately before or after surgery when they are likely to be in a more anxious, distressed, or cognitively impaired state from sedatives or anesthetics. From an ethical standpoint, this is important with regard to adequacy of informed consent. Second, communication is improved with the intraoperative anesthesia team when there is sufficient time for concerns of all parties to be elicited, discussed, and clarified. Finally, this early encounter and assessment affords time to prepare for and enact management plans for specific therapies.

Opioid Agonists

The anesthesiologist must first determine which patients require extra attention and should be considered opioid tolerant. Tolerance is defined by the Food and Drug Administration (FDA) as the use of greater than or equal to 60 mg of oral morphine equivalents per day for 7 days or longer, regardless of long-term opioid use.[5] Opioid-tolerant patients may be taking a variety of opioids at home in immediate-release, short-acting (eg, oxycodone, hydrocodone, morphine, oral transmucosal fentanyl) or extended-release, long-acting (eg, morphine sulfate [MS Contin], oxycodone hydrochloride [OxyContin], transdermal fentanyl patch) preparations. Routes of administration may include oral, subcutaneous, transdermal, or intrathecal delivery. Patients should be advised to continue their usual analgesic regimen, including regularly scheduled immediate- or extended-release and transdermal agents.

Methadone is a mu-receptor opioid agonist that may be prescribed for the treatment of chronic pain or as a once-daily opioid replacement therapy for addiction. These patients have tolerance to opioids but may also have increased pain sensitivity.[13] Patients on methadone for both chronic pain or methadone maintenance therapy should continue their scheduled regimen perioperatively to avoid fluctuations in methadone levels given its long half-life.[13,14]

An evidence-based multimodal analgesic plan is necessary for opioid-tolerant patients to provide adequate analgesia and prevent withdrawal but also to reduce the length of hospital stay and prevent occurrences of readmission.[5] Despite the FDA definition of tolerance, in clinical acute pain practice, chronic use of relatively low levels of daily opioid exposure (20 mg morphine equivalents daily for greater than 7–10 days) can significantly reduce the effectiveness of postoperative opioids, leading to poorly controlled pain.

The specific components of any multimodal analgesic plan will vary based on specific patient and surgical factors, but includes regional or neuraxial anesthesia/analgesia when possible, nonopioid adjunct agents (eg, nonsteroidal antiinflammatory drugs [NSAIDs]/cyclooxygenase-2 [COX-2] inhibitors, acetaminophen, gabapentinoids, alpha-agonists, intravenous [IV] lidocaine), and NMDA-receptor antagonists (eg, ketamine), using opioids for rescue analgesia only. Preoperative dosing of nonopioid analgesics is gaining popularity and typically involves medications taken before surgery and continued around-the-clock postoperatively (**Table 1**). Pregabalin,[15–18] gabapentin, and celecoxib[19] have demonstrated benefit when started preoperatively in reducing the need for postoperative opioids. The combination of acetaminophen, pregabalin, and celecoxib has shown benefit when started preoperatively and continued around-the-clock postoperatively.[20] At the authors' institution, this has been adopted for orthopedic, urologic, and gynecologic procedures.

Table 1		
Multimodal nonopioid agents for preemptive analgesia		
Drug	**Administration Route**	**Suggested Dose (2 h Before Surgery)**
Acetaminophen	PO	1000 mg (more than 50 kg)
Celecoxib	PO	200–400 mg
Pregabalin	PO	75–150 mg
Gabapentin	PO	900–1200 mg

INTRAOPERATIVE MANAGEMENT

In the PSH model, the anesthesiologist caring for patients on the day of surgery will have the advantage of the thorough preoperative assessment and management strategy already in place. The anesthesiologist can then advise patients of the finalized anesthetic plan. Patients should continue their analgesic regimen up until the time of surgery, including any morning doses of opioid.

While tailoring the analgesic plan, the anesthesiologist must also take into account the nature of patients' pain and the mechanisms of analgesic agents to be used. Pain is complex and subjective; there are 5 generally recognized categories of pain: nociceptive, neuropathic, psychogenic, mixed, and idiopathic[21]:

- Nociceptive pain can be described as sharp or dull, aching, throbbing, pressure-like, or feelings of stiffness.
- Neuropathic pain is often burning, shocklike tingling, or stabbing.
- Mixed pain is a result of stimulation of both nociceptive and neuropathic pathways.
- Psychogenic pain is pain that is thought to be an emotional or psychiatric phenomenon, only to be considered once all other nociceptive or neuropathic causes have been ruled out.
- Idiopathic pain is due to unknown origin.

The concept of multimodal analgesia takes into account understanding the type of pain in need of treatment and targeting it at multiple sites along the pain pathway to achieve a synergistic effect with different classes of analgesics.

- Opioids act both supraspinally via inhibitory pathways as well as in the dorsal horn to impede nociception.
- NSAIDs act both in the spinal cord and periphery, inhibiting cyclooxygenase to decrease inflammation secondary to prostaglandins and further decrease nociception.
- Acetaminophen acts centrally likely via inhibition of cyclooxygenase in treating nociceptive pain.
- Local anesthetics act at central, spinal, and peripheral sites, depending on route or localization of administration.
- NMDA receptor antagonists, exerting effects in the dorsal horn, inhibit nociceptive and neuropathic pain.
- Gabapentinoids bind to calcium channels in the spinal cord and brain to decrease neuropathic pain.

Although opioid-tolerant patients presenting for surgery will need opioids perioperatively, multimodal pain regimens are paramount in managing acute surgical pain in these cases. These regimens may include the use of intraoperative adjuncts, such as epidural/regional analgesia, ketamine, dexmedetomidine, and lidocaine infusions.

Ketamine

A single dose of opioid will lead to activation of NMDA receptors.[22] In theory, tolerance and hyperalgesia begins with the first dose of an opioid. In animal studies, ketamine, an NMDA-receptor antagonist, reversed morphine tolerance and improved effectiveness while additionally preventing acute tolerance.[23] The use of ketamine as an analgesic adjunct in opioid-naïve patients resulted in decreased opioid requirements after surgery; fewer opioid-related side effects, such as nausea and vomiting; and possibly prevention of chronic pain and hyperalgesia.[24–26] Few studies, however, have examined the effect of intraoperative ketamine in opioid-tolerant patients.

A study by Loftus and colleagues[27] showed that intraoperative ketamine infusions resulted in reduced opioid requirements in the first 48 hours and at 6 weeks postoperatively in opioid-dependent patients undergoing back surgery. Additionally, average pain scores were significantly reduced in the postanesthesia care unit (PACU) and at 6 weeks postoperatively.[27] The investigators recommended patients taking 30 mg or more per day of morphine equivalents with expected moderate-severe postsurgical pain receive a bolus of ketamine of 0.5 mg/kg followed by infusion of 0.25 mg/kg/h intraoperatively.

Postoperatively, ketamine infusions may be safely administered without continuous cardiac or respiratory monitoring (intensive care unit or telemetry).[28] An in-house acute pain management service (APMS) team is crucial to provide regular monitoring of analgesia and titration. Although studies demonstrate that it is well tolerated, patients should be monitored for neurologic and psychological side effects.

Regional Anesthesia and Analgesia

Several surgical procedures, including extremity surgery, carotid endarterectomy, and hernia repair, may be done under a regional/neuraxial block as the sole anesthetic, thus decreasing the reliance of opioids in opioid-tolerant patients.

Although general anesthesia is often indicated, regional analgesia as part of a multimodal regimen decreases opioid burden in these challenging patients. The use of long-acting local anesthetics and continuous catheters enable regional analgesia to be effective during the first few days following surgery when acute pain is most severe.

Utilization of perineural catheters results in prolonged postoperative pain control (including resting and dynamic pain), accelerated resumption of therapy, less reliance on opioids, fewer sleep disturbances, and overall increased patient satisfaction.[29] Epidural analgesia results in improved rehabilitation, better pain control, and decreased opioid consumption when compared with opioids alone.[30]

Appropriate regional techniques, including single-shot or continuous peripheral nerve blocks or epidural analgesia, should be used whenever possible. Although regional anesthesia offers many benefits in opioid-tolerant patients, opioids must be judiciously continued to prevent withdrawal and to treat the chronic pain not related to the surgical procedure.

Lidocaine Infusions

The use of an IV lidocaine infusion has been widely studied in abdominal surgery. In open and laparoscopic abdominal surgery, an IV lidocaine infusion resulted in decreased postoperative pain for 48 hours postoperatively, reduced opioid consumption, earlier return of bowel function, earlier rehabilitation, and decreased length of stay.[31]

When compared with thoracic epidural analgesia in patients undergoing colorectal surgery, intraoperative and postoperative lidocaine infusions resulted in similar times to return of bowel function and time to discharge; however, epidural analgesia resulted in lower numeric pain scores.[32]

The benefit of intraoperative lidocaine infusions may not apply to all types of surgery as the addition of lidocaine in patients undergoing mastectomy did not result in decreased pain or reduced opioid consumption when compared with placebo.[33] Although the use of intraoperative lidocaine infusions has not been well studied in the opioid-tolerant population, current literature suggests it may be useful as part of a multimodal regimen when regional techniques are contraindicated. A common dosing strategy is a 1.5-mg/kg loading dose followed by 1.5 mg/kg/h intraoperatively.

Dexmedetomidine

With the high density of receptors in the dorsal horn, alpha-2 adrenergic agonists act on the central nervous system to reduce pain. Dexmedetomidine is a highly selective alpha-2 agonist that acts as a sedative, anxiolytic, sympatholytic, and analgesic with minimal respiratory depression.

In rats with presumed neuropathic pain, dexmedetomidine exhibited antihyperalgesic action.[34] In patients undergoing laparoscopic bariatric surgery, randomized to receive 0.2, 0.4, or 0.8 mcg/kg/h dexmedetomidine infusion intraoperatively, dexmedetomidine decreased opioid use, need for antiemetic treatment, and length of stay in the PACU but did not change opioid use patterns or quality of recovery beyond the PACU.[35]

Given the cardiovascular effects of dexmedetomidine infusions, namely, bradycardia and hypotension, Tufanogullari and colleagues[35] recommended a 0.2-mcg/kg/h infusion intraoperatively as an analgesic adjunct. Gurbet and colleagues[36] showed an intraoperative dexmedetomidine rate of 0.5 mcg/kg/h decreased 48-hour opioid consumption with no change in pain scores following total abdominal hysterectomy when compared with placebo. Although dexmedetomidine has not been specifically studied in the opioid-tolerant population, the literature suggests a continuous infusion during surgery may decrease intraoperative opioid requirements. It is likely that continuation of dexmedetomidine is necessary to extend opioid reduction beyond the PACU.

POSTOPERATIVE MANAGEMENT

The care of opioid-tolerant patients continues well beyond the operating room and into the PACU as part of the PSH model. Although the surgeon typically orders analgesics for the patients when on the medical ward, there is substantial opportunity for input and collaboration by the anesthesiologist. Medication management and expectations for postoperative analgesia can be established early on and can help create a positive patient experience.

In this section, strategies to managing postoperative analgesia for opioid-tolerant patients are discussed, including

- Benefits of a nonopioid multimodal approach
- Resuming home medications, including opioid agonist-antagonists
- The role of acute pain services in the PSH model

Multimodal Approach to Postoperative Analgesia

Inadequate postoperative pain management has been linked with complications, including myocardial ischemia, impaired pulmonary function, ileus, thromboembolism, impaired immune function, wound infection, and anxiety.[37] Additionally, hospital reimbursements are now linked to patient satisfaction scores (Hospital Consumer Assessment of Healthcare Providers and Systems [HCAHPS]). Pain is a significant driver of poor patient satisfaction. Poor outcomes related to uncontrolled pain result in greater health care costs.

Multimodal analgesia has been successfully implemented into multiple surgical pathways, and has been shown to reduce opioid consumption,[38] surgical complications,[38,39] and length of hospital stay.[38–40] Some agents that have been used successfully in multimodal pathways include acetaminophen (by mouth and IV), COX-2 inhibitors, gabapentinoids (gabapentin and pregabalin), NSAIDs, glucocorticoids, local anesthetics, α-2 agonists (clonidine and dexmedetomidine), and ketamine (**Table 2**). To the extent possible, these agents can be used to minimize opioids and improve analgesia.

Table 2
Multimodal nonopioid agents for postoperative analgesia

Drug	Administration Route	Suggested Dose and Frequency
Acetaminophen	PO/IV	1000 mg q 6 h (more than 50 kg)
Ibuprofen	PO	600 mg q 6 h
Ketorolac	PO/IV	15–30 mg q 6 h
Celecoxib	PO	200–400 mg q 12 h
Gabapentin	PO	600–800 mg TID
Pregabalin	PO	75–150 mg q 12 h
Ketamine	IV	0.5 mg/kg bolus; infusion 0.25 mg/kg/h

Multimodal analgesia pathways have existed for more than 15 years; but Kehlet and colleagues[41] were the first to describe pathways leading to clinically important outcomes, such as reduction in length of hospital stay in colorectal procedures. There have been several large reviews and meta-analyses summarizing the literature on several multimodal agents, with both gabapentin[42] and pregabalin[43] demonstrating an opioid-reducing effect when used in a multimodal pathway. The addition of an NSAID to an opioid as part of a multimodal pathway provides better analgesia than the opioid alone.[44] Taken together, these studies provide evidence that using nonopioid agents whenever possible can improve analgesia; this is even more so for opioid-tolerant patients.

Because the doses of opioids taken chronically by the opioid-tolerant population often exceed many physicians' comfort levels, surgeons frequently seek recommendations on discharge regimens. Conversion from IV to oral opioids requires experience and expertise of a physician experienced in pain management.[45]

Postoperative Oral Analgesics and Restarting Home Medications

If patients were taking a combination opioid preoperatively (eg, hydrocodone/acetaminophen), that creates an opportunity for the anesthesiologist to initiate a discussion with the surgeon about postoperative analgesics. Nonopioid adjuncts, such as acetaminophen, NSAIDs, and gabapentinoids, should be initiated as the mainstay of treatment, with opioids for breakthrough pain only. Unless patients underwent gastrointestinal surgery or cannot take anything by mouth for other reasons, oral medications may be started on the evening of the day of surgery. However, for patients admitted to the hospital after painful surgery, IV opioids are often needed. Opioids delivered via IV patient-controlled analgesia (PCA) lead to better patient satisfaction than intermittent boluses given via oral, intramuscular, or IV routes as well as lower rates of adverse events.[46] More potent opioids, such as hydromorphone or sufentanil, may be considered when treating opioid-tolerant patients. Higher-dose PCA settings may be needed to deliver adequate analgesia.

SPECIAL CONSIDERATIONS: OPIOID ADDICTION THERAPY

Patients treated for opioid addiction present a particular challenge in that many have a history of longstanding opioid abuse with significant tolerance and hyperalgesia. It is not unusual for patients in recovery to be exceedingly fearful of exposure to nonmaintenance opioids if they are on such a regimen, or reexposure to opioids if they have managed to be fully abstinent. In addition to the opioid agonist methadone, patients being treated with opioid-replacement therapy (ORT) may be maintained on buprenorphine (categorized as a partial agonist, although its pharmacology is debated) or an opioid antagonist (naltrexone), each with unique considerations.

Buprenorphine

Buprenorphine is a semisynthetic opioid with a high mu-receptor binding affinity. It is marketed as a sole agent (Subutex) or in combination with naloxone (Suboxone) to deter abuse. A transbuccal patch delivery form of buprenorphine has been recently approved by the FDA for the treatment of chronic pain, There are limited data to guide perioperative management of patients taking buprenorphine; furthermore, its high binding affinity, slow dissociation, and analgesic ceiling effect may make adequate analgesia a challenge.

Analgesic strategies for patients on buprenorphine mainly stem from expert opinion and case reports. Bryson[13] describes 2 basic treatment options as continuing buprenorphine throughout the perioperative period or stopping buprenorphine before surgery.

There is no clear consensus on the best strategy for managing buprenorphine preoperatively, with many recommending it be stopped preoperatively to avoid the analgesic ceiling effect of buprenorphine or the high dose of supplemental opioids that may be required. Discontinuation of ORT, however, carries a risk of relapse that will need to be evaluated on an individual patient basis. Considering the high prevalence of substance abuse and addiction in the United States, involving consultants with addiction medicine expertise on perioperative teams may be a useful approach going forward.

In patients for whom the medication is discontinued preoperatively, it should be stopped 3 days before surgery. As long as the drug has been given sufficient time to be metabolized by the liver and excreted by the biliary system (typically 72 hours), mu-opioid agonists may be effectively used for postoperative analgesia, taking into account that most of these patients are opioid tolerant and require larger-than-standard doses. Although the duration of action for buprenorphine is about 40 hours,[47] the elimination half-life after a sublingual dose is 37 hours.[48] If buprenorphine-naloxone was given within the preceding 3 days before surgery, its effects may still be present as it has a very strong binding affinity for the mu-opioid receptor and dissociates very slowly from the receptor.[47] If opioids are used for postoperative analgesia, the resulting analgesia may not be adequate using routine clinical doses if some of the buprenorphine is still present because of competitive binding of buprenorphine and its ceiling effect. Emphasis should be on regional anesthesia techniques and nonopioid agents, especially ketamine as a potent analgesic that does not affect respiratory drive[49] and provides the most benefit after painful procedures.[50]

For patients who continue taking buprenorphine-naloxone through the perioperative period, buprenorphine can provide sufficient and potent opioid analgesia as a partial mu-opioid agonist and for minor procedures may be adequate without much supplementation.[13] For major surgery, however, additional analgesics will likely be needed. One investigator recommends the use of short-acting opioids, such as fentanyl, if a once-daily dosing regimen of buprenorphine-naloxone is continued perioperatively,[13] though he noted that higher doses might be required. Additional doses of buprenorphine are often sufficient to manage pain within a multimodal analgesic regimen. Trying to overpower the effect of buprenorphine with other opioids may provide unpredictable results as well as unpredictable opioid side effects. For upper- or lower-extremity surgery, peripheral nerve blocks can often eliminate the need for supplemental opioids. A multimodal strategy will help minimize opioids. Early involvement by an APMS is recommended.

In the absence of definitive recommendations, the anesthesiologist will help decide whether to discontinue or continue the buprenorphine preoperatively, possibly in conjunction with the prescribing physician who should be involved with postdischarge planning and management. It cannot be emphasized enough how important collaboration and coordination are for safe and effective perioperative care of this complicated patient population.

Naltrexone

In contrast to buprenorphine or methadone, naltrexone is a full opioid competitive antagonist used in the treatment of opioid and alcohol addiction and is available as a once-daily oral agent or a monthly depot injection (Vivitrol). Overcoming the competitive blockade with opioid agonists to achieve analgesia requires markedly high doses of opioid medications and is not recommended. With the plasma half-life of oral naltrexone at 4 hours, and that of the active metabolite at 13 hours, patients should be advised not to take their once-daily dose on the morning of surgery.[13] With the monthly depot injection, the antagonism lasts roughly 30 days; elective surgery should be delayed until at least 30 days after the last naltrexone injection if possible.[13]

Patients treated for opioid addiction benefit from a preoperative plan regarding management of antagonist/mixed agents but may present for surgery, either emergently or having bypassed preoperative assessment, without such a plan. A careful discussion among patients, the anesthesiologist, and the surgical team is important, as opioids will be less effective or even ineffective in the setting of these agents. A decision will need to be made to proceed, maximizing nonopioid medications in a multimodal strategy, or to delay surgery.

The recommendations for managing postoperative analgesia for patients taking buprenorphine-naloxone through the perioperative period undergoing moderately or severely painful surgery are summarized as follows:

- Incorporate regional anesthesia techniques whenever possible.
- Administer nonopioid adjuncts unless contraindicated.
- If opioids are used, higher doses may be needed, the analgesic effect may be less, and the resulting side effects greater, justifying appropriately increased levels of monitoring.
- Consider involving an APMS early.

Acute Pain Management Services in the Perioperative Surgical Home

The postoperative period presents an excellent opportunity for an anesthesiologist-led APMS to actively help guide patients through hospitalization until discharge and beyond. Delivering patients safely through the intraoperative period is no longer sufficient. Adequate postoperative analgesia is a key area within the PSH that has an impact on long-term outcomes for patients. In the case of opioid-tolerant patients, the postoperative period is frequently the most challenging. Careful planning may yield significant improvements for these patients.

Continuous peripheral nerve blocks have continued to increase in popularity, especially in opioid-tolerant patients.[51] The APMS has an important role in managing continuous peripheral nerve blocks and providing patient education. At the authors' institution, the APMS physicians and colleagues skilled in regional anesthesia techniques work together to manage these patients who received a peripheral nerve block, including providing 24-hour coverage via a beeper that patients may call for problems or questions. Regional anesthesia and analgesic techniques will likely become even more important as their inclusion in surgical pathways increases.[45]

A summary of the benefits of an APMS in the perioperative surgical home in the setting of opioid-tolerant patients in the postoperative period is as follows:

- Management of continuous peripheral nerve blocks, including titration, side effects, and ambulatory catheter instructions, from the recovery room until discharge and beyond
- Initiation and management of adjunctive medications, such as ketamine, that require expertise beyond the typical analgesic regimen
- Guidance and recommendations on opioid conversions and discharge regimens that include high opioid doses

SUMMARY

Management of acute pain with minimization of adverse events in opioid-tolerant patients undergoing surgery can be extremely challenging. The anesthesiologist, using his or her expertise in regional anesthesia techniques and pharmacology, can improve patient care within the PSH by implementing a comprehensive opioid-reducing strategy for opioid-tolerant patients that begins in the early preoperative period. Intraoperative care of these patients relies heavily on a multimodal analgesic regimen to minimize required opioids, and a postoperative APMS may help transition from the hospital setting to discharge. Anesthesiologists are expected to be involved in the entire perioperative process. Challenging patients, such as the opioid tolerant, demand our expertise, especially as the specialty of anesthesiology evolves to perioperative medicine.

For those practitioners working in institutions without discrete acute pain services or perioperative surgical home, a good place to start is to initiate discussions with the quality assessment and performance improvement team to bring these issues to the forefront. Interested practitioners can also approach their anesthesia and surgical colleagues to spark initiatives. Collaboration with anesthesia departments at other institutions that have implemented some elements of the PSH can be extremely helpful, especially with administrative or financial concerns. Changing institutional culture is difficult, and individual champions for improvement can be confronted by resentment if they take these issues on alone.

Future study will be needed to demonstrate the efficacy of the PSH, but the benefits seen by similar programs and the support of the ASA give optimism. The Triple Aim requires not only anesthesiologist expertise but also collaboration with physician colleagues and hospital administration. Through continued improvement measures, anesthesiologists are positioned to greatly improve the perioperative continuum.

REFERENCES

1. Gan TJ, Habib AS, Miller TE, et al. Incidence, patient satisfaction, and perceptions of post-surgical pain: results from a US national survey. Curr Med Res Opin 2014;30:149–60.
2. Kain Z, Vakharia S, Garson L, et al. The perioperative surgical home as a future perioperative practice model. Anesth Analg 2014;118(5):1126–30.
3. Berwick DM, Nolan TW, Whittington J. The triple aim: care, health, and cost. Health Aff 2008;27:759–69.
4. Vetter TR, Boudreaux AM, Jones KA, et al. The perioperative surgical home: how anesthesiology can collaboratively achieve and leverage the triple aim in health care. Anesth Analg 2014;118(5):1131–6.
5. Abel RB, Rosenblatt MA. Preoperative evaluation and preparation of patients for orthopedic surgery. Anesthesiol Clin 2014;32:881–92.

6. Gulur P, Williams L, Chaudhary S, et al. Opioid tolerance – a predictor of increased length of stay and higher readmission rates. Pain Physician 2014;17: E503–7.

7. Institute of Medicine (US) Committee on Advancing Pain Research, Care, and Education. Relieving pain in America: a blueprint for transforming prevention, care, education, and research. Washington, DC: National Academies Press; 2011.

8. Mahathanaruk M, Hitt J, de LeonCasasola OA. Perioperative management of the opioid tolerant patient for orthopedic surgery. Anesthesiol Clin 2014;32:923–32.

9. Angst M. Intraoperative use of remifentanil for TIVA: postoperative pain, acute tolerance, and opioid-induced hyperalgesia. J Cardiothorac Vasc Anesth 2015; 29(Suppl 1):S16–22.

10. Kim SH, Stoicea N, Soghomonyan S, et al. Intraoperative use of remifentanil and opioid induced hyperalgesia/acute opioid tolerance: systematic review. Front Pharmacol 2014;5:108.

11. Lee M, Silverman S, Hansen H, et al. A comprehensive review of opioid-induced hyperalgesia. Pain Physician 2011;14:145–61.

12. Yi P, Pryzbylkowski P. Opioid induced hyperalgesia. Pain Med 2015;16:S32–6.

13. Bryson E. The perioperative management of patients maintained on medications used to manage opioid addiction. Curr Opin Anaesthesiol 2014;27:359–64.

14. Peng PWH, Tumber PS, Gourlay D. Review article: perioperative pain management of patients on methadone therapy. Can J Anaesth 2005;52(5):513–23.

15. Bornemann-Cimenti H, Lederer AJ, Wejbora M, et al. Preoperative pregabalin administration significantly reduces postoperative opioid consumption and mechanical hyperalgesia after transperitoneal nephrectomy. Br J Anaesth 2012; 108:845–9.

16. Buvanendran A, Kroin JS, Della Valle CJ, et al. Perioperative oral pregabalin reduces chronic pain after total knee arthroplasty: a prospective, randomized, controlled trial. Pain Med 2010;110(1):199.

17. Sawan H, Chen AF, Viscusi ER, et al. Pregabalin reduces opioid consumption and improves outcome in chronic pain patients undergoing total knee arthroplasty. Phys Sportsmed 2014;42(2):10–8.

18. Kim JC, Choi YS, Kim KN, et al. Effective dose of peri-operative oral pregabalin as an adjunct to multimodal analgesic regimen in lumbar spinal fusion surgery. Spine 2011;36(6):428–33.

19. Derry S, Moore RA. Single dose oral celecoxib for acute postoperative pain in adults. Cochrane Database Syst Rev 2013;(10):CD004233.

20. Trabulsi EJ, Patel J, Viscusi ER, et al. Preemptive multimodal pain regimen reduces opioid analgesia for patients undergoing robotic-assisted laparoscopic radical nephrectomy. Urology 2010;76(5):1122–4.

21. Welchek CM, Mastrangelo L, Sinatra RS, et al. Qualitative and quantitative assessment of pain. In: Sinatra R, de Leon-Cassasola OA, Ginsberg B, et al, editors. Acute pain management. New York: Cambridge University Press; 2009. p. 147–66.

22. Larcher A, Laulin JP, Celerier E, et al. Acute tolerance associated with a single opiate administration: involvement f N-methyl-D-aspartate-dependent pain facilitatory systems. Neuroscience 1998;84(2):583–9.

23. Shimoyama N, Shimoyama M, Inturrisi CE, et al. Ketamine attenuates and reverses morphine tolerance in rodents. Anesthesiology 1996;85:1357–66.

24. Laulin JP, Marette P, Corcuff JB, et al. The role of ketamine in preventing fentanyl-induced hyperalgesia and subsequent acute morphine tolerance. Anesth Analg 2001;94(5):263–9.

25. Subramaniam K, Subramaniam B, Steinbrook RA. Ketamine as adjuvant analgesic to opioids: a quantitative and qualitative systematic review. Anesth Analg 2004;99(2):482–95.

26. Bell RF, Dahl JB, Moore RA, et al. Perioperative ketamine for acute postoperative pain. Cochrane Database Syst Rev 2006;(1):CD004603.

27. Loftus RW, Yeager MP, Clark JA, et al. Intraoperative ketamine reduces perioperative opiate consumption in opiate-dependent patients with chronic back pain undergoing back surgery. Pain Med 2010;113:639–46.

28. Schwenk ES, Baratta JL, Gandhi K, et al. Setting up an acute pain management service. Anesthesiol Clin 2014;32:893–910.

29. Ilfeld BM. Continuous peripheral nerve blocks: a review of the published evidence. Anesth Analg 2011;113(4):904–25.

30. Capdevila X, Berthelet Y, Biboulet P, et al. Effects of perioperative analgesic technique on the surgical outcome and duration of rehabilitation after major knee surgery. Anesthesiology 1999;91(1):8–15.

31. McCarthy GC, Megalla SA, Habib AS. Impact of intravenous lidocaine infusion on postoperative analgesia and recovery from surgery: a systematic review of randomized controlled trials. Drugs 2010;70(9):1149–63.

32. Wongyingsinn M, Baldini G, Charlebois P, et al. A randomized controlled trial in patients undergoing laparoscopic colorectal surgery using an enhanced recovery program. Reg Anesth Pain Med 2011;36:241–8.

33. Terkawi AS, Durieux ME, Gottschalk A, et al. Effect of intravenous lidocaine on postoperative recovery of patients undergoing a mastectomy: a double-blind, placebo-controlled randomized trial. Reg Anesth Pain Med 2014;39(6):472–7.

34. Poree LR, Guo TZ, Kingery WS, et al. The analgesic potency of dexmedetomidine is enhanced after nerve injury: a possible role for peripheral alpha2-adrenoreceptors. Anesth Analg 1998;87:941–8.

35. Tufanogullari B, White PF, Peixoto MP, et al. Dexmedetomidine infusion during laparoscopic bariatric surgery: the effect on recovery outcome variables. Anesth Analg 2008;106(6):1741–8.

36. Gurbet A, Basagan-Mogol E, Turker G, et al. Intraoperative infusion of dexmedetomidine reduces perioperative analgesic requirements. Can J Anaesth 2006; 53(7):646–52.

37. Joshi GP, Ogunnaike BO. Consequences of inadequate postoperative pain relief and chronic persistent postoperative pain. Anesthesiol Clin North America 2005; 23:21–36.

38. Larson DW, Lovely JK, Cima RR, et al. Outcomes after implementation of a multimodal standard care pathway for laparoscopic colorectal surgery. Br J Surg 2014;101:1023–30.

39. Madani A, Fiore JF, Wang Y, et al. An enhanced recovery pathway reduces duration of stay and complications after open pulmonary lobectomy. Surgery 2015; 158:899–910.

40. Michelson JD, Addante RA, Charlson MD. Multimodal analgesia therapy reduces length of hospitalization in patients undergoing fusions of the ankle and hindfoot. Foot Ankle Int 2013;34:1526–34.

41. Kehlet H, Jensen TS, Woolf CJ. Persistent postsurgical pain: risk factors and prevention. Lancet 2006;367:1618–25.

42. Hurley RW, Cohen SP, Williams KA, et al. The analgesic effects of perioperative gabapentin on postoperative pain: a meta-analysis. Reg Anesth Pain Med 2006;31:237–47.
43. Zhang J, Ho KY, Wang Y. Efficacy of pregabalin in acute postoperative pain: a meta-analysis. Br J Anaesth 2011;106:454–62.
44. Elia N, Lysakowski C, Tramer MR. Does multimodal analgesia with acetaminophen, nonsteroidal antiinflammatory drugs, or selective cyclooxygenase-2 inhibitors and patient-controlled analgesia morphine offer advantages over morphine alone? Anesthesiology 2005;103:1296–304.
45. Walters TL, Mariano ER, Clark JD. Perioperative surgical home and the integral role of pain medicine. Pain Med 2015;16:1666–72.
46. Viscusi ER. Patient-controlled drug delivery for acute postoperative pain management: a review of current and emerging technologies. Reg Anesth Pain Med 2008;33:146–58.
47. Chen KY, Chen L, Mao J. Buprenorphine-naloxone therapy in pain management. Anesthesiology 2014;120:1262–74.
48. Elkader A, Sproule B. Buprenorphine: clinical pharmacokinetics in the treatment of opioid dependence. Clin Pharmacokinet 2005;44:661–80.
49. Craven R. Ketamine. Anaesthesia 2007;62:48–53.
50. Laskowski K, Stirling A, McKay WP, et al. A systematic review of intravenous ketamine for postoperative analgesia. Can J Anaesth 2011;58:911–23.
51. Rapp SE, Ready LB, Nessly ML. Acute pain management in patients with prior opioid consumption: a case-controlled retrospective review. Pain 1995;61:195–201.

Can Chronic Pain Be Prevented?

Ignacio J. Badiola, MD[a,b],*

KEYWORDS

- Chronic pain • Persistent postsurgical pain • Acute to chronic pain transition
- Genetics of chronic pain • Multimodal analgesia

KEY POINTS

- Acute pain is an important and appropriate warning system signaling danger to an individual. This pain can persist and become chronic, often serving no further potentially beneficial function, leading to suffering. The pathophysiology behind this transition is under investigation, and significant advances in understanding of the role acute pain has on the development of chronic pain have been made over the past 20 years.
- Although all chronic pain is at one point acute, it is difficult in many chronic pain conditions to identify the precise time point of the beginning of pain. Chronic pain after surgery can serve as a framework for the study of the mechanisms and risk factors of transition to chronic pain because the precise timing of the injury can be identified.
- Various agents and therapeutic options for treating acute pain are available; however, larger randomized clinical trials are needed to identify their role in preventing the transition to chronic pain after surgery.

INTRODUCTION

All patients who undergo a surgical procedure or suffer a traumatic event have some form of acute pain from tissue injury. In most, this acute pain associated with the tissue injury subsides over a short period as the tissue heals. Many patients, however, continue to complain—and suffer—after the "normal" healing process has taken place. Persistent postsurgical pain (PPSP) serves as a framework for studying the development of chronic pain because the precise timing of the injury can be identified.[1] PPSP is an important public health problem with a prevalence approximating the prevalence of chronic pain.[2,3] Patients who experience PPSP may have pain severe enough to interfere with almost every aspect of life, including sleep, mood, work, and social life, which is common in other forms of chronic pain.

[a] Department of Anesthesiology and Critical Care, Perelman School of Medicine, University of Pennsylvania, Philadelphia, PA, USA; [b] Penn Pain Medicine Center, 1840 South Street, Philadelphia, PA 19146, USA
* Penn Pain Medicine Center, 1840 South Street, Philadelphia, PA 19146.
E-mail address: Ignacio.badiola@uphs.upenn.edu

Anesthesiology Clin 34 (2016) 303–315
http://dx.doi.org/10.1016/j.anclin.2016.01.008
anesthesiology.theclinics.com
1932-2275/16/$ – see front matter © 2016 Elsevier Inc. All rights reserved.

Macrae[4] proposed a working definition of PPSP as pain that should have developed after the surgical procedure and has been present for at least 2 months. Other causes of pain, including pain from a preexisting problem, must first be excluded.

This review begins by looking at the common surgical procedures known to be associated with a high incidence of PPSP. The mechanisms involved in the transition from acute to chronic pain after surgery are reviewed and current understanding on halting the transition by exploiting these mechanisms discussed. Risk factors involved, including medical, psychological, and genetic factors, are assessed. This article concludes by evaluating various treatment options that are at the disposal of anesthesiologists and surgeons.

COMMON SURGICAL PROCEDURES ASSOCIATED WITH PERSISTENT POSTSURGICAL PAIN

Persistent Pain After Breast Surgery

Persistent pain after breast surgery is a clinical problem that affects between 25% and 50% of patients.[5] There are many surgical procedures (lumpectomy, mastectomy, and axillary node dissection) as well as nonsurgical procedures (radiation and chemotherapy) that are usually done in conjunction with surgery.[6] Risk factors proposed include younger age, preoperative pain in other locations, axillary lymph node dissection (compared with sentinel lymph node biopsy or no axillary intervention), radiotherapy, and nerve lesioning.[6] Heterogeneity in current studies makes it difficult to draw conclusions with regard to diagnosis and treatment. Only a few studies have reviewed possible risk factors using a prospective design, adding to the difficulty.[7] Many of the studies did not use current surgical/adjuvant therapy and there are inconsistencies in how chronic pain is defined as well as how preoperative, intraoperative, and postoperative data were collected.[6]

Thoracic Surgery

The incidence of chronic pain after thoracotomy is estimated at 30% to 50%. Injuries to the intercostal nerve by incision, rib retraction, placement of trocars, and suturing are all possible mechanisms[8] and seem to be some of the most important factors.[9] Various groups have evaluated classic risk factors of PPSP after thoracic surgery (ie, preoperative pain, acute pain severity, gender, age, and psychosocial factors) as well as classic factors associated with PPSP in cancer surgery, such as radiation and chemotherapy, with variable results.[9] There are various surgical approaches to performing a thoracotomy, including a posterolateral approach, anterior approach, and a muscle-sparing posterolateral approach. The latter 2 approaches are muscle sparing and may allow for better visualization of the ribs. Khan and colleagues[10] compared a muscle-sparing thoracotomy with a traditional posterolateral approach in 10 patients and noted no difference in chronic pain. Another study looking at 335 patients (148 patients in the muscle-sparing group and 187 in traditional thoracotomy) noted no difference in frequencies of chronic pain 1 year after surgery.[11] An anterior limited thoracotomy may have some benefit in PPSP compared with a posterolateral thoracotomy; however, this result was from a retrospective trial with only 28 patients in each group.[12]

Video-assisted thoracic surgery is a minimally invasive approach that spares the long incision of a thoracotomy. The belief is that small incisions may eliminate nerve injury. Although there is some evidence of this in retrospective studies, prospective studies do not conclude any benefit. Preoperative and postoperative patient factors and missing surgical details preclude any conclusion at to the benefit of video-assisted thoracic surgery in reducing PPSP.[9] There are few studies evaluating analgesic techniques, such as thoracic epidural analgesia, paravertebral blocks, intercostal blocks, and interpleural analgesia, precluding any recommendations regarding these techniques. A critical review by Wildgaard and colleagues[9] notes that future studies should focus on prospective trials (most have been retrospective) and should have more detailed preoperative, intraoperative, and postoperative data, especially on nerve handling with objective assessment of nerve function.

Postamputation Phantom Limb Pain

The incidence of PPSP after amputation ranges from 50% to 85%.[4] This is significant when considering that more than 185,000 upper or lower extremity amputations are done yearly.[13] Pain is considered secondary to a combination of nociceptive and neuropathic mechanisms.[14] Pain is classified as phantom limb pain or residual limb pain (stump pain). Nonpainful sequela include phantom sensations. A systematic review from 2002 looked at preoperative and postoperative interventions, including regional nerve blocks, epidural, calcitonin, and transcutaneous electrical nerve stimulation unit. There was significant limitations with the studies themselves, including poor quality and contradictory results.[15] Another systematic review for amputation from peripheral vascular disease evaluated 11 studies using various agents, including local anesthetics, opiates, N-methyl-D-aspartate (NMDA) antagonists, α_2-agonists, and γ-aminobutyric acid analogs in various combinations and in various techniques (epidural, oral, intravenous, and perineural) and also concluded that there is a lack of evidence supporting the use of preemptive analgesia in minimizing chronic pain after amputation.[16]

MECHANISMS FOR THE DEVELOPMENT OF PERSISTENT POSTSURGICAL PAIN

In the past 10 to 15 years, many advances in the understanding of the acute to chronic pain transition have been elucidated at the cell and molecular levels. The complete picture, however, is not yet understood. It seems, however, that abnormal changes in the nociceptive process, especially with regard to continuation of the sensitization that occurs after tissue injury, play an important role. Central sensitization is a prolonged increase in the excitability and synaptic efficacy of neurons involved in central nociceptive pathways.[17] Sensitization transpires in both the peripheral nervous system and central nervous system (CNS), with changes occurring in neurons as well as the supporting cells, such as glial and immune cells.

The initial injury occurs in the periphery (ie, with the incision), leading to primary hyperalgesia. This injury results in release of inflammatory mediators, which act on nociceptor terminals. Activation of various intracellular pathways ultimately leads to changes in the threshold and kinetics of the nociceptor.[18] The immune system is also involved, with neutrophil and macrophages drawn to the site of tissue damage. These immune cells release various factors, such as interleukin and tumor necrosis factor (TNF)-α. The release of TNF-α may increase the release of metalloproteinases,[19] leading to breakdown of the blood nerve barrier, allowing macrophages access to the dorsal root ganglion. These changes are important for the development of central sensitization.

Central sensitization presents as hyperalgesia, pain hypersensitivity, tactile allodynia, punctate/pressure hyperalgesia, and enhanced temporal summation.[17] As in peripheral sensitization, neuronal, glial, and immune cells are involved. Afferent barrage of peripheral nociceptors to the dorsal horn produces an increase in the spatial extent of the cutaneous receptive fields of dorsal horn neurons, amplifies the response of these neurons, and reduces their thresholds.[20] The CNS then reacts more so than before the injury to the same input from the periphery. Neuronal cells in the dorsal horn recruit NMDA receptors that bind glutamate, a major excitatory amino acid. Binding of glutamate leads to increases in intracellular calcium levels with subsequent depolarization and neuronal excitement. Many other pathways with multiple mediators are involved in central sensitization, including substance P, calcitonin gene-related peptide, and sarcoma family kinases.[18] Together, these pathways cause a more robust response by the CNS to the peripheral input than there is if no central sensitization is present. The sustained input from the periphery to the CNS causes changes in gene transcription in the dorsal root ganglion, leading to an enhancement in neuronal excitability, which persists.[21] Changes in the activity of the dorsal horn neuron depends on a balance between excitatory and inhibitory input from supraspinal centers, and imbalance can render the dorsal horn neurons more sensitive. The 2 commonly studied supraspinal centers are the serotonergic pathway via the rostral ventromedial medulla and the noradrenergic efferent from the locus ceruleus. The catecholamine released from the cerulospinal pathway acts on α_2-adrenergic receptors inhibiting excitatory neurotransmitter release.[22] Proteases, such as cathepsin G, are up-regulated in the dorsal horn after surgery. In rat models, inhibiting cathepsin G decreased chronic inflammation associated hyperalgesia with a resultant decrease in neutrophilic infiltration and lower levels of interleukin 1β in the dorsal horn.[23] These investigators also looked at 246 patients with PPSP and noted that variations in the cathepsin G gene were associated with a decrease in risk of PPSP.[23]

The immune system is important in both peripheral and central sensitization. At the location of injury, neutrophils and macrophages are attracted to and release mediators, including prostaglandins and cytokines, such interleukin 6, TNF-α, and leukemia inhibitory factor. These mediators recruit further macrophages to the site of injury. The blood nerve barrier is broken down, allowing macrophages into the dorsal horn. Sprouting of sympathetic nerve fibers around the dorsal horn contributes to neuropathic pain.[18] Peripheral nerve injury leads to activation of microglia, astrocytes, and other immune cells in the CNS. Microglia switch into a state or reactive gliosis. Unrestrained gliosis may sustain central sensitization.[24] The immune system has also been implicated in opioid-induced hyperalgesia. In a rat study, inducing hyperalgesia with morphine was reversed by ablating spinal microglia while not affecting morphine-induced antinociception.[25]

Genetics also plays a major role because polymorphisms in genes are involved in increasing or decreasing the risk. Agents or techniques that potentiate or inhibit the mediators that result from these genes may play a role in decreasing the risk of developing chronic pain. More research on the development of new biomarkers and analgesics are needed to both treat and predict PPSP.[22]

GENETICS/EPIGENETICS OF PERSISTENT POSTSURGICAL PAIN

Not all patients with the same classic risk factors undergoing the same procedure go on to develop PPSP, leading to the likelihood that individual risk factors, especially genetic determinants, may play a role. Hereditability provides the ability to compare the relative importance of genetic and nongenetic (ie, environmental) influence on the variation of traits within and across a population.[26] Current genetic studies estimate that heritability is approximately 50% in chronic pain. Chronic pain in general, and PPSP in particular, is a complex disorder with many genetic variants combining to influence the risk of transitioning from an acute to a chronic pain state.[27] The simplest mutations involve single-nucleotide polymorphisms, a variation in a single nucleotide of an allele that can affect function of the product of that gene. Other mutations involve changes that are more complex in sequence. Genes that code for proteins involved in ion channels, receptors, transporters, transcription factors, and hormone receptors have been identified and may be involved in PPSP.[27] For example, the CACNG2 gene encodes a protein involved in trafficking AMPA receptors and possibly a calcium channel subunit and affects susceptibility to chronic pain after nerve injury. In a study of 549 breast cancer patients who underwent a unilateral mastectomy, of whom 215 reported chronic pain, 5 of 12 single-nucleotide polymorphism haplotype tests performed showed association with chronic pain individually.[28]

P2X7R codes for the P2X7 receptor, an ionotropic ATP-gated receptor. Some mutations in this gene are associated with less mechanical allodynia and nerve injury–induced pain behaviors in mice. In humans, a cohort of postmastectomy patients and patients with osteoarthritis showed lower pain intensities if they carried the (hypofunctional) P2X7R allele.[29]

Currently, several investigators are looking at the genetics of various chronic pain disease states: The Orofacial Pain: Prospective Evaluation and Risk Assessment project is evaluating the genetics behind temporomandibular pain[30–32]; the fibromyalgia family study has evaluated familial aggregation of fibromyalgia,[33] and the arcOGEN consortium and other investigators have looked at the genetics of osteoarthritis.[34–36]

Although the genetic makeup of an individual contributes to the genotype of an individual, not all with the same genotype develop the same phenotype. More than 99.9% of the human genome is identical between individuals,[37] with only 0.1% of genes contributing to the variability seen among humans.[38] This 0.1% difference, however, is not enough to explain differences in pain perception between individuals. For example, monozygotic twins can still develop different pain phenotypes. The environment plays a key role in shaping the pain phenotype of an individual. Epigenetics studies how a change in genetic makeup is not required to produce a different phenotype (ie, how individuals with the same genotype have varying phenotypes).[39] Factors, such as stress and the psychosocial environment, affect the susceptibility of an individual to developing persistent pain by means of DNA sequence–independent mechanisms. Epigenetic regulation directs the way genes are expressed based on environmental conditions.[40] These environmental factors were noted to play a role in the development of neck pain in twins[41] as well as response to opioids.[42] Mechanistically, these environmentally mediated changes involve histone acetylation, RNA interference, and DNA methylation.[38] The field of epigenetics in chronic pain continues to unfold, and how it will affect the ability to curtail the transmission to PPSP is still unknown.

RISK FACTORS FOR THE DEVELOPMENT OF CHRONIC PAIN AFTER SURGERY

Each patient who ultimately goes on to develop PPSP has a specific medical history, belief system, psyche, and genotype that together determine risk. Classic risk factors include preoperative pain experiences, exposures and current levels, high postoperative pain intensity, age, gender, genetics, intraoperative nerve injury, and psychosocial factors.[21,43] **Box 1** summarizes these factors. Not all these variables, however, lead to chronic pain when present. For example, intraoperative nerve injury is a known risk factor for developing chronic pain; however, only 10% of patients undergoing mandibular osteotomy with known nerve injury go on to develop chronic pain.[44]

Deumans and colleagues[22] have described these risk factors as vulnerability factors. The ideal model for studying the development of PPSP would include both preoperative and postoperative assessment of psychological and neuropsychological

---

Box 1
Risk factors for the development of postoperative pain

- Gender (female)
- Age (younger)
- Preoperative pain at surgical site
- Preoperative pain at site other than surgical site
- Exaggerated response to experimental pain stimuli
- Anxiety
- Catastrophizing
- Depression
- Lack of support in patient's environment
- Surgical fear
- Lower income
- Poor preoperative quality of life
- Lower education level
- Preoperative analgesic use
- Specific genetics/genotype
- Redo surgery
- Site of surgery (mastectomy, amputation, thoracotomy, hernia)
- Large versus a small surgical incision
- Intraoperative nerve damage
- Postoperative severe pain
- High postoperative analgesic use
- Radiation therapy
- Chemotherapy
- Stress

---

factors, detailed intraoperative data on the handling of tissues and nerves, detailed early and late postoperative pain data, and a thorough clinical investigation to exclude other causes of chronic pain states.[43]

Younger age in adults is a consistent risk factor associated with the development of PPSP,[4,7,43,45–47] but this is not universal.[3,48] Gender is important, with most studies noting a higher risk in female patients compared with male patients.[47,49] One theory is that sex hormones and other sex related mechanisms are important in the activation of glial cells needed for the development of central sensitization.[18]

One of the most consistent risk factors is the intensity of acute postoperative pain.[50–52] This seems to occur across surgery types and regardless of time frame.[46] Given the mechanisms of PPSP development, this makes biological sense. Postoperative pain creates a barrage of input from the periphery to the CNS. It activates the CNS, causing peripheral and central sensitization, leading to neuroplastic changes. One trigger thought to induce pain chronicity is the amount of injury-related discharge during surgery and its impact on the CNS.[46] Although it may seem obvious to avoid nerve injury, this may not be possible in certain procedures, such as amputation. More commonly, smaller nerves are inadvertently injured while cutting skin, muscle, fascia, and bone.

Psychosocial factors are important, with some investigators suggesting that they may be more important than medical factors.[53,54] Preoperative anxiety, catastrophizing, depression, stress, late return to work, and psychological vulnerability showed correlation with PPSP.[54,55] Not all studies looking at specific psychological variables arrive at the same conclusion. Powell and colleagues[56] evaluated patients at 4 months after inguinal hernia surgery and found that lower preoperative optimism was a risk factor whereas other emotional variables were not. There is significant heterogeneity of psychological studies making it difficult to formulate a meta-analysis. For example, Hinrichs-Rocker and colleagues'[54] systematic review noted that some studies assessed prediction variables and outcome variables using standard measurements whereas others used surrogate endpoints. Recommendations for future studies included the use of standardized instruments to collect data (ie, State-Trait Anxiety Inventory).[54] Larger prospective studies permitting more powerful multivariate analysis are needed. Results should include intercorrelation between predictors and more uniform outcome measures that allow statistical pooling.[55]

ANALGESIA FOR PREVENTION OF CHRONIC PAIN

Analgesia used in the perioperative setting is based on the assumption that disrupting peripheral and central sensitization lowers the risk of developing chronic pain. As discussed previously, the transition to chronic pain involves many pathways and mediators, and many analgesics in current use exploit these pathways. Not all analgesic methods are associated with clinically important disruption of sensitization, however, and, therefore, may have limited impact on the risk of developing chronic pain.

Nonsteroidal Anti-inflammatory Drugs

Nonsteroidal anti-inflammatory drugs (NSAIDS) decrease prostaglandin synthesis by inhibiting cyclooxygenase (COX). There are at least 2 isoforms of COX—COX-1 and COX-2—with COX-2 more important in inflammation. There are 3 prospective randomized trials that are heterogeneous, differing in NSAID used, follow-up time point, and pain outcomes, with none showing any significant impact on incidence or severity of PPSP.[57] Two of these trials evaluated ibuprofen on chronic pain after mastectomy and the other trial evaluated parecoxib on mammoplasty. Based on these 3 trials, NSAIDS cannot be recommended for PPSP risk reduction.

Gabapentin

Gabapentin inhibits calcium inflow and excitatory neurotransmitter release by binding to the $\alpha 2\delta$ subunit of presynaptic voltage-gated calcium channels. A review in 2011 found 10 clinical trials evaluating varying doses, timing, length of treatment, and surgeries.[58] Five of the studies had data evaluating any pain at 3 months and none showed any difference in the development of PPSP over placebo. Similarly, none of the studies noted any difference in PPSP development from placebo at 6 months. Only 2 studies of the 6, however, reported the primary outcome of that systematic review: incidence of any pain. This systematic review concluded that gabapentin failed to show any benefit over placebo in reducing PPSP. Nevertheless, the total sample size of these studies was small (133 receiving gabapentin and 147 placebo). The longest administration was 30 days postoperatively, with many studies providing only a single dose preoperatively or postoperatively. It is still too early to make a definitive case for gabapentin. Future studies should focus on more standardized doses on more homogeneous surgical populations. The length of administration should take into account the expected length of the entire period of acute postoperative pain and continued for that period.[1]

Pregabalin

Pregabalin's mechanism of action is similar to that of gabapentin. Evaluating pregabalin for PSPP also presents a problem due to heterogeneity of available studies. Six studies have evaluated pregabalin at various doses, timing/duration of treatment, and surgery type. These six studies include cardiac surgery, total knee arthroplasty, lumbar discectomy, major spine surgery, and thyroidectomy.[59–65] Five of these studies were systematically reviewed by Chapparo and colleagues,[58] concluding that at 3 months pregabalin was substantially better than placebo in reducing the proportion of participants reporting any pain at the anatomic site of the procedure or pain referred to the surgical site (their primary outcome) in only 1 study.[63] A more recent study of pregabalin for off-pump coronary artery bypass graft procedures did not show a benefit of pregabalin in reducing chronic pain at 3 months.[65] One trial noted reduction of chronic neuropathic pain at 3 months and 6 months after total knee arthroplasty.[62] The only study looking at patients for 12 months did not show any benefit of pregabalin over placebo in reducing PPSP.[60] Like gabapentin, it is still too early to make a conclusion on whether pregabalin makes any difference in preventing PPSP.

Ketamine

Ketamine is an NMDA receptor antagonist. This receptor plays a role in central sensitization. A review of 14 trials looking at various dosages and administration times noted significant differences in how long and when ketamine was administered.[58] Six of the studies used a total dose of less than 1 mg/kg, 4 studies between 1 mg/kg and 2 mg/kg, and 4 studies more than a total of 2 mg/kg. Five studies evaluated incidence of pain at 3 months (thoracotomy, breast, orthopedic, and hernia surgery). The overall risk ratio showed no effect of ketamine over placebo in PPSP prevention.[58] A subgroup of these patients, however, who received ketamine for longer than 24 hours indicated an advantage of ketamine over placebo. Eight of the 14 trials evaluated the incidence of PPSP at 6 months. These were also in a heterogeneous surgical population (joint replacement surgery, amputation surgery, thoracotomy, mixed orthopedic surgery, rectal carcinoma resection, and breast surgery and radical prostatectomy). Ketamine was superior to placebo. A subgroup analysis showed that this was the case only for ketamine treatment less than 24 hours. Nevertheless, another systematic review and meta-analysis concluded that there was no benefit of ketamine in reducing chronic pain.[14,66] Since Chaparro and colleagues review, no ketamine trials have evaluated the use of ketamine in preventing PPSP.[57] The heterogeneity in surgery types, dosing, and administration timing enables making a definitive conclusion about ketamine difficult.

Regional Anesthesia/Neuroaxial Anesthesia

Regional anesthesia is one of the most effective tools in decreasing acute postoperative pain. In doing so, it may decrease the barrage of input to the CNS, thus reducing central sensitization and possibly PPSP. In animal models, regional anesthesia was shown to help block postsurgical sensitization and pain vulnerability; however, this was negated when high-dose fentanyl was used intraoperatively.[67] Andreae and colleagues[68] performed an analysis on 1090 patients with outcomes reported at 6 months and 441 patients reported at 12 months. Pooled data favored epidural placement for thoracotomy (based on 250 patients) and paravertebral blocks for breast cancer surgery at 6 months (based on 89 patients), leading them to conclude that epidural anesthesia may decrease the risk of PPSP after thoracotomy in 1 of 4 patients, and paravertebral blocks applied in breast cancer surgery seem to reduce this risk in 1 of 5 patients. The investigators caution that these results are based on studies that have several shortcomings, including heterogeneity, attrition, and incomplete data.[68] Many of the studies evaluating regional anesthesia have demonstrated better pain relief acutely but have not provided conclusive evidence in decreasing PPSP.[21] Many of these studies have significant heterogeneity biases, including multiple nerve blocks, differences in regional anesthetic techniques, and various surgical procedures.

Multimodal Analgesia

Multimodal therapy involves combinations of techniques and pharmacologic agents to target pain along various pathways that influence transduction, transmission, and modulation of nociceptive signals.[69] Evidence shows a multimodal approach may decrease use of opioid and reduce opioid-related adverse effects in the perioperative period. Although promising in its perioperative use for pain management, there have been limited trials looking at how multimodal therapy in the perioperative period changes PPSP outcomes. A regimen of gabapentin, eutectic mixture of local anesthetics cream, and ropivacaine in the wound during breast cancer surgery was compared with placebo with significant improvement in both pain and analgesia use at months and 6 months postoperatively.[70] Clarke and colleagues[57] noted 2 multimodal analgesia trials with 1 study showing benefit at 3 months and the other at 1 year postoperatively. Further well-controlled studies looking at various multimodal regimens in various surgical procedures are needed to draw firm conclusions regarding the use of multimodal analgesia in preventing PPSP.

SUMMARY

Chronic pain that develops after a surgical insult is hypothesized to at least in part be due to nerve injury or from central sensitization. Minimizing that nerve damage or preventing central sensitization should theoretically reduce the chronification of pain.[1] Recently, an Initiative on Methods, Measurement, and Pain Assessment in Clinical Trials meeting took place with experts from diverse government agencies, universities, industry, and countries.[1] Their focus was to facilitate the identification of preventative interventions and design of clinical trials for the prevention of chronic pain. Some of their recommendations include beginning treatment prior to the pain-causing event, such that the effective dose is present before surgery. This may take weeks or months. The agent/intervention should be continued, if possible, for the entire period of acute postoperative pain, which can be many months, depending on the surgical procedure. This may be more difficult in interventions that rely on intravenous or regional anesthetic techniques but should be less of a problem for oral medications, such as gabapentin and pregabalin.

Significant strides in understanding the mechanism, risk factors, and treatment strategies in the transition to chronic pain have been made over the past 20 years, yet much remains to be discovered. Significant limitations exist in the current literature to make concrete recommendations for specific patients undergoing specific surgical procedures. Desperately needed are large-scale, multicenter, randomized trials. Collaboration between scientists and clinicians is vital as new biological acumen into the genetics and molecular mechanisms of acute to chronic pain transitions are elucidated.

REFERENCES

1. Gewandter JS, Dworkin RH, Turk DC, et al. Research design considerations for chronic pain prevention clinical trials: IMMPACT recommendations. Pain 2015; 156:1184–97.
2. Kalso E. IV. Persistent post-surgery pain: research agenda for mechanisms, prevention, and treatment. Br J Anaesth 2013;111:9–12.
3. Johansen A, Romundstad L, Nielsen CS, et al. Persistent postsurgical pain in a general population: prevalence and predictors in the Tromso study. Pain 2012; 153:1390–6.
4. Macrae WA. Chronic post-surgical pain: 10 years on. Br J Anaesth 2008;101: 77–86.
5. Gartner R, Jensen MB, Nielsen J, et al. Prevalence of and factors associated with persistent pain following breast cancer surgery. JAMA 2009;302:1985–92.
6. Andersen KG, Kehlet H. Persistent pain after breast cancer treatment: a critical review of risk factors and strategies for prevention. J Pain 2011;12:725–46.
7. Andersen KG, Duriaud HM, Jensen HE, et al. Predictive factors for the development of persistent pain after breast cancer surgery. Pain 2015;156(12):2413–22.
8. Elmore B, Nguyen V, Blank R, et al. Pain management following thoracic surgery. Thorac Surg Clin 2015;25:393–409.
9. Wildgaard K, Ravn J, Kehlet H. Chronic post-thoracotomy pain: a critical review of pathogenic mechanisms and strategies for prevention. Eur J Cardiothorac Surg 2009;36:170–80.
10. Khan IH, McManus KG, McCraith A, et al. Muscle sparing thoracotomy: a biomechanical analysis confirms preservation of muscle strength but no improvement in wound discomfort. Eur J Cardiothorac Surg 2000;18:656–61.
11. Landreneau RJ, Pigula F, Luketich JD, et al. Acute and chronic morbidity differences between muscle-sparing and standard lateral thoracotomies. J Thorac Cardiovasc Surg 1996;112:1346–50 [discussion: 1350–1].
12. Nomori H, Horio H, Suemasu K. Anterior limited thoracotomy with intrathoracic illumination for lung cancer: its advantages over anteroaxillary and posterolateral thoracotomy. Chest 1999;115:874–80.
13. Hsu E, Cohen SP. Postamputation pain: epidemiology, mechanisms, and treatment. J Pain Res 2013;6:121–36.
14. Humble SR, Dalton AJ, Li L. A systematic review of therapeutic interventions to reduce acute and chronic post-surgical pain after amputation, thoracotomy or mastectomy. Eur J Pain 2015;19:451–65.
15. Halbert J, Crotty M, Cameron ID. Evidence for the optimal management of acute and chronic phantom pain: a systematic review. Clin J Pain 2002;18:84–92.
16. Ypsilantis E, Tang TY. Pre-emptive analgesia for chronic limb pain after amputation for peripheral vascular disease: a systematic review. Ann Vasc Surg 2010;24: 1139–46.
17. Woolf CJ. Central sensitization: implications for the diagnosis and treatment of pain. Pain 2011;152:S2–15.
18. Mifflin KA, Kerr BJ. The transition from acute to chronic pain: understanding how different biological systems interact. Can J Anaesth 2014;61:112–22.

19. Shubayev VI, Angert M, Dolkas J, et al. TNFalpha-induced MMP-9 promotes macrophage recruitment into injured peripheral nerve. Mol Cell Neurosci 2006; 31:407–15.
20. Woolf CJ, King AE. Dynamic alterations in the cutaneous mechanoreceptive fields of dorsal horn neurons in the rat spinal cord. J Neurosci 1990;10:2717–26.
21. Richebe P, Julien M, Brulotte V. Potential strategies for preventing chronic post-operative pain: a practical approach: continuing professional development. Can J Anaesth 2015;62(12):1329–41.
22. Deumens R, Steyaert A, Forget P, et al. Prevention of chronic postoperative pain: cellular, molecular, and clinical insights for mechanism-based treatment approaches. Prog Neurobiol 2013;104:1–37.
23. Liu X, Tian Y, Meng Z, et al. Up-regulation of cathepsin G in the development of chronic postsurgical pain: an experimental and clinical genetic study. Anesthesiology 2015;123:838–50.
24. Grace PM, Hutchinson MR, Maier SF, et al. Pathological pain and the neuroimmune interface. Nat Rev Immunol 2014;14:217–31.
25. Ferrini F, Trang T, Mattioli TA, et al. Morphine hyperalgesia gated through microglia-mediated disruption of neuronal Cl(-) homeostasis. Nat Neurosci 2013;16:183–92.
26. Visscher PM, Hill WG, Wray NR. Heritability in the genomics era–concepts and misconceptions. Nat Rev Genet 2008;9:255–66.
27. Clarke H, Katz J, Flor H, et al. Genetics of chronic post-surgical pain: a crucial step toward personal pain medicine. Can J Anaesth 2015;62:294–303.
28. Nissenbaum J, Devor M, Seltzer Z, et al. Susceptibility to chronic pain following nerve injury is genetically affected by CACNG2. Genome Res 2010;20:1180–90.
29. Sorge RE, Trang T, Dorfman R, et al. Genetically determined P2X7 receptor pore formation regulates variability in chronic pain sensitivity. Nat Med 2012;18:595–9.
30. Smith SB, Mir E, Bair E, et al. Genetic variants associated with development of TMD and its intermediate phenotypes: the genetic architecture of TMD in the OPPERA prospective cohort study. J Pain 2013;14:T91–101.
31. Slade GD, Fillingim RB, Sanders AE, et al. Summary of findings from the OPPERA prospective cohort study of incidence of first-onset temporomandibular disorder: implications and future directions. J Pain 2013;14:T116–24.
32. Smith SB, Maixner DW, Greenspan JD, et al. Potential genetic risk factors for chronic TMD: genetic associations from the OPPERA case control study. J Pain 2011;12:T92–101.
33. Arnold LM, Fan J, Russell IJ, et al. The fibromyalgia family study: a genome-wide linkage scan study. Arthritis Rheum 2013;65:1122–8.
34. Hudson G, Panoutsopoulou K, Wilson I, et al. No evidence of an association between mitochondrial DNA variants and osteoarthritis in 7393 cases and 5122 controls. Ann Rheum Dis 2013;72:136–9.
35. Elliott KS, Chapman K, Day-Williams A, et al. Evaluation of the genetic overlap between osteoarthritis with body mass index and height using genome-wide association scan data. Ann Rheum Dis 2013;72:935–41.
36. arcOGEN Consortium, arcOGEN Collaborators, Zeggini E, et al. Identification of new susceptibility loci for osteoarthritis (arcOGEN): a genome-wide association study. Lancet 2012;380:815–23.
37. International HapMap Consortium. The international hapmap project. Nature 2003;426:789–96.
38. Kim H, Dionne RA. Individualized pain medicine. Drug Discov Today Ther Strateg 2009;6:83–7.

39. Buchheit T, van de Ven T, Shaw A. Epigenetics and the transition from acute to chronic pain. Pain Med 2012;13:1474–90.
40. Bai G, Ren K, Dubner R. Epigenetic regulation of persistent pain. Transl Res 2015;165:177–99.
41. Fejer R, Hartvigsen J, Kyvik KO. Heritability of neck pain: a population-based study of 33,794 Danish twins. Rheumatology (Oxford) 2006;45:589–94.
42. Angst MS, Phillips NG, Drover DR, et al. Pain sensitivity and opioid analgesia: a pharmacogenomic twin study. Pain 2012;153:1397–409.
43. Kehlet H, Jensen TS, Woolf CJ. Persistent postsurgical pain: risk factors and prevention. Lancet 2006;367:1618–25.
44. Jaaskelainen SK, Teerijoki-Oksa T, Virtanen A, et al. Sensory regeneration following intraoperatively verified trigeminal nerve injury. Neurology 2004;62: 1951–7.
45. Joris JL, Georges MJ, Medjahed K, et al. Prevalence, characteristics and risk factors of chronic postsurgical pain after laparoscopic colorectal surgery: retrospective analysis. Eur J Anaesthesiol 2015;32:712–7.
46. Katz J, Seltzer Z. Transition from acute to chronic postsurgical pain: risk factors and protective factors. Expert Rev Neurother 2009;9:723–44.
47. Peng Z, Li H, Zhang C, et al. A retrospective study of chronic post-surgical pain following thoracic surgery: prevalence, risk factors, incidence of neuropathic component, and impact on qualify of life. PLoS One 2014;9:e90014.
48. Hoofwijk DM, Fiddelers AA, Peters ML, et al. Prevalence and predictive factors of chronic postsurgical pain and poor global recovery one year after outpatient surgery. Clin J Pain 2015;31(12):1017–25.
49. Reddi D, Curran N. Chronic pain after surgery: pathophysiology, risk factors and prevention. Postgrad Med J 2014;90:222–7 [quiz: 226].
50. VanDenKerkhof EG, Hopman WM, Goldstein DH, et al. Impact of perioperative pain intensity, pain qualities, and opioid use on chronic pain after surgery: a prospective cohort study. Reg Anesth Pain Med 2012;37:19–27.
51. Steyaert A, De Kock M. Chronic postsurgical pain. Curr Opin Anaesthesiol 2012; 25:584–8.
52. Shipton EA. The transition from acute to chronic post surgical pain. Anaesth Intensive Care 2011;39:824–36.
53. Block AR, Ohnmeiss DD, Guyer RD, et al. The use of presurgical psychological screening to predict the outcome of spine surgery. Spine J 2001;1:274–82.
54. Hinrichs-Rocker A, Schulz K, Jarvinen I, et al. Psychosocial predictors and correlates for chronic post-surgical pain (CPSP) - a systematic review. Eur J Pain 2009; 13:719–30.
55. Theunissen M, Peters ML, Bruce J, et al. Preoperative anxiety and catastrophizing: a systematic review and meta-analysis of the association with chronic postsurgical pain. Clin J Pain 2012;28:819–41.
56. Powell R, Johnston M, Smith WC, et al. Psychological risk factors for chronic postsurgical pain after inguinal hernia repair surgery: a prospective cohort study. Eur J Pain 2012;16:600–10.
57. Clarke H, Poon M, Weinrib A, et al. Preventive analgesia and novel strategies for the prevention of chronic post-surgical pain. Drugs 2015;75:339–51.
58. Chaparro LE, Smith SA, Moore RA, et al. Pharmacotherapy for the prevention of chronic pain after surgery in adults. Cochrane Database Syst Rev 2013;(7):CD008307.
59. Suehs BT, Louder A, Udall M, et al. Impact of a pregabalin step therapy policy among medicare advantage beneficiaries. Pain Pract 2014;14:419–26.

60. Gianesello L, Pavoni V, Barboni E, et al. Perioperative pregabalin for postoperative pain control and quality of life after major spinal surgery. J Neurosurg Anesthesiol 2012;24:121–6.
61. Burke SM, Shorten GD. Perioperative pregabalin improves pain and functional outcomes 3 months after lumbar discectomy. Anesth Analg 2010;110:1180–5.
62. Buvanendran A, Kroin JS, Della Valle CJ, et al. Perioperative oral pregabalin reduces chronic pain after total knee arthroplasty: a prospective, randomized, controlled trial. Anesth Analg 2010;110:199–207.
63. Pesonen A, Suojaranta-Ylinen R, Hammaren E, et al. Pregabalin has an opioid-sparing effect in elderly patients after cardiac surgery: a randomized placebo-controlled trial. Br J Anaesth 2011;106:873–81.
64. Kim SY, Jeong JJ, Chung WY, et al. Perioperative administration of pregabalin for pain after robot-assisted endoscopic thyroidectomy: a randomized clinical trial. Surg Endosc 2010;24:2776–81.
65. Joshi SS, Jagadeesh AM. Efficacy of perioperative pregabalin in acute and chronic post-operative pain after off-pump coronary artery bypass surgery: a randomized, double-blind placebo controlled trial. Ann Card Anaesth 2013;16: 180–5.
66. Klatt E, Zumbrunn T, Bandschapp O, et al. Intra- and postoperative intravenous ketamine does not prevent chronic pain: a systematic review and meta-analysis. Scand J Pain 2015;7:42–54.
67. Meleine M, Rivat C, Laboureyras E, et al. Sciatic nerve block fails in preventing the development of late stress-induced hyperalgesia when high-dose fentanyl is administered perioperatively in rats. Reg Anesth Pain Med 2012;37:448–54.
68. Andreae MH, Andreae DA. Local anaesthetics and regional anaesthesia for preventing chronic pain after surgery. Cochrane Database Syst Rev 2012;10: CD007105.
69. Gritsenko K, Khelemsky Y, Kaye AD, et al. Multimodal therapy in perioperative analgesia. Best Pract Res Clin Anaesthesiol 2014;28:59–79.
70. Fassoulaki A, Triga A, Melemeni A, et al. Multimodal analgesia with gabapentin and local anesthetics prevents acute and chronic pain after breast surgery for cancer. Anesth Analg 2005;101:1427–32.

Interventional Treatments of Cancer Pain

Jill E. Sindt, MD*, Shane E. Brogan, MB BCh

KEYWORDS

- Cancer pain • Intrathecal drug delivery • Vertebroplasty • Kyphoplasty • Neurolysis
- Celiac plexus • Superior hypogastric plexus • Ganglion impar

KEY POINTS

- Intrathecal drug delivery should be considered for patients with cancer experiencing opioid-related side effects or pain refractory to opioid dose escalation.
- In cancer patients with painful vertebral compression fractures that have failed to improve with conservative treatment, vertebral augmentation is a safe and minimally invasive technique that improves both pain and function.
- Neurolysis of the celiac plexus, superior hypogastric plexus, or ganglion impar is indicated in patients with cancer with visceral upper abdominal, lower abdominal, or perineal pain, respectively.
- Radiofrequency ablation and cryoablation are safe and effective techniques for the management of isolated painful bony metastases.

INTRODUCTION

Pain is a ubiquitous experience for patients with cancer, affecting more than 90% of patients during their treatment. In greater than half of all patients with advanced cancer it remains at least moderately severe. Cancer-related pain is associated with reduced ability to tolerate treatment, depression, and diminished quality of life and is demoralizing to patients and caregivers.[1] Although the use of opioids for cancer pain remains a mainstay in accordance with the World Health Organization's analgesic ladder, this approach does not produce adequate pain control in an estimated 20% to 30% of patients.[2,3]

Interventional techniques have been proposed as the "fourth step" in the analgesic ladder, appropriate for patients in whom pain is refractory to systemic opioids.[4] In addition there is growing recognition of the role of interventional procedures early in the course of cancer-related pain to avoid unnecessary suffering and morbidity.[5]

Disclosures: Dr J.E. Sindt has served as a consultant for Medtronic, Inc, Langhorne, PA. Dr S.E. Brogan has served as a speaker and consultant for Medtronic, Inc, Langhorne, PA. Department of Anesthesiology, University of Utah School of Medicine, 30 North 1900 East Room C3444, Salt Lake City, UT 84132, USA
* Corresponding author.
E-mail address: Jill.Sindt@hsc.utah.edu

However, interventional procedures remain underutilized in clinical practice because of unfamiliarity with these procedures and lack of qualified interventional pain specialists.[6] This article reviews interventional treatments for cancer pain, including technique, indications, complications, and outcomes.

INTRATHECAL DRUG DELIVERY

Intrathecal drug delivery (IDD) entails the administration of drugs, typically opioids with or without adjunct medications, directly to the cerebrospinal fluid and to the central nervous system receptor sites via a subarachnoid catheter. The analgesic agent is delivered from an implanted device or, less commonly, an external pump. Because IDD allows the drug to largely bypass the systemic circulation, it results in minimal systemic side effects, yet superior analgesia, at a fraction of the comparable systemic dose. Furthermore, IDD allows for direct access to central nervous system receptors, bypassing issues of drug absorption from the gastrointestinal tract and first pass metabolism, permitting analgesic efficacy of drugs that would be otherwise toxic, such as local anesthetics and novel peptides like ziconotide.

Indications

- Cancer-related pain refractory to systemic opioids despite dose escalation
- Dose-limiting opioid side effects
- Inability of patients with cancer-related pain to safely use systemic opioids; for example, patients with severe medical comorbidities, a history of opioid addiction or active drug use.

Pharmacologic Options

Opioids are the most commonly used medications in IDD; however, multiple other medications have been used safely and effectively. **Table 1** summarizes the mechanism, indications, and adverse effects of these agents.

Methods of Intrathecal Drug Delivery

Percutaneous catheter
The simplest delivery system involves a catheter inserted into the intrathecal space percutaneously and then connected to an external infusion pump. Advantages of percutaneous catheters include ease of insertion or removal, ability to titrate medications quickly, and ability for providers who are not pain specialists to manage symptoms in the home. Disadvantages include limited longevity (days to weeks), infectious risk, catheter disconnections, interference with patient mobility, and need to frequently change the medication solution in the external pump.

Presently, in the United States, there are no products specifically approved for percutaneous intrathecal use, though an epidural catheter can easily be used for this purpose.

Implanted drug delivery systems
In this method of IDD, a small electronic pump is placed subcutaneously in the anterior abdominal wall and connected to a catheter that is tunneled subcutaneously around the abdomen and inserted into the intrathecal space in the lumbar spine (**Fig. 1**). The pump has a reservoir that can be refilled percutaneously using a port that is accessed by a needle through the skin. The advantages of IDD systems (IDDS) include low maintenance, less infectious risk, lack of interference with patient mobility, and durability of the system. Disadvantages include the need for surgical procedure and general anesthesia, access to an experienced pain provider for pump placement

Table 1
Pharmacotherapy for IDD

Drug	Mechanism	Indications	Adverse Effects	Notes
Morphine Hydromorphone Fentanyl Sufentanil	Mu-agonists	First-line therapy for nociceptive or mixed pain Second-line therapy for neuropathic pain	Sedation, nausea, pruritus, respiratory depression, urinary retention	Morphine is FDA approved for intrathecal delivery Fentanyl and sufentanil are typically added as second opioid or after failure of initial opioid
Ziconotide (Prialt)	N-type calcium channel blockade	First-line or second-line therapy for nociceptive and neuropathic pain	Mood disturbance, visual hallucinations, ataxia, elevated creatine kinase	FDA approved for intrathecal delivery
Bupivacaine	Sodium channel blockade	First-line therapy for neuropathic pain; second-line therapy for nociceptive pain	Motor weakness, urinary retention, hypotension, bradycardia	Typically used in combination with an opioid
Clonidine	Alpha-2 agonist	Third-line therapy for nociceptive or neuropathic pain	Ataxia, sedation, bradycardia, postural hypotension	Serious withdrawal syndrome with abrupt discontinuation
Baclofen	Central-acting GABA-agonist	Third-line therapy for nociceptive or neuropathic pain, especially if spasticity is present	Motor weakness, bradycardia, hypotension	Potentially fatal withdrawal syndrome with abrupt discontinuation

Abbreviations: FDA, Food and Drug Administration; GABA, γ-aminobutyric acid.
Data from Refs.[7–9]

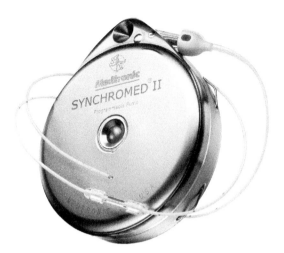

Fig. 1. IDDS. (*Reprinted* with the permission of Medtronic, Inc. © 2014.)

and management, high initial costs, and the logistics of returning to the clinic regularly for pump refills and programming changes. Currently in the United States there are 3 available implantable IDDS: the SynchroMed II (Medtronic Inc, Langhorne, PA), the Codman 3000 (Codman and Shurtleff, Inc, Raynham, MA), and the Prometra (Flowonix Medical Inc, Mount Olive, NJ). However, the SynchroMed II is the most commonly used among these, owing to its larger available reservoir sizes (20 mL and 40 mL), ability to program complex dose schedules, and inclusion of a remote-control device to allow for the administration of patient-controlled boluses for the management of breakthrough pain.

Complications of Intrathecal Drug Delivery

Most complications with IDD are technical in nature and associated with the procedural insertion; however, complications with the implanted or externalized pump and intrathecal catheter have also been reported (**Table 2**).[10,11]

Efficacy of Intrathecal Drug Delivery for Cancer Pain

Multiple studies have demonstrated the success of IDD, reporting improved pain control, increased survival, fewer side effects, reduced opioid use, and potentially lower cost (for long-surviving patients) as compared with treatment with systemic opioids.[7,8,12–16]

- A 2002 study by Smith and colleagues[13] randomized 202 patients with advanced cancer to medical management or IDDS plus medical management. At 4 weeks the IDDS group had lower pain scores, lower toxicity scores, and reduced rates of fatigue and sedation.[12] In 2005, the same group reported on the 6-month follow-up of these patients and reported that IDDS reduced pain scores and analgesic-related toxicity and was associated with increased survival.
- Burton and colleagues[14] in 2004 published a study of neuraxial analgesia in which 56 patients with refractory cancer pain were treated with IDD for 8 weeks with reduced pain scores, reduced drowsiness, reduced oral opioid use, and a significant reduction in the proportion of patients with severe pain (86% to 17%).
- In 2015 Brogan and colleagues[15] published a prospective study of 58 patients who received IDDS for refractory cancer pain, noting improvements in pain scores, symptom severity scores, and symptom interference scores as well

Table 2
Technical complications associated with intrathecal drug delivery

Complication	Symptoms	Management
Superficial skin infection	Erythema along incision	Oral or IV antibiotics, rarely system must be removed
Pump pocket infection	Erythema or drainage from incision, pocket erythema or tenderness, possible systemic symptoms (fever, chills, malaise)	Must remove pump; catheter often removed; antibiotics per cultures
Pump pocket seroma/hematoma	Swelling and palpable fluid around pump pocket	Abdominal binder, warm compresses; may require ultrasound-guided drainage of fluid
Meningitis	Headache, nuchal rigidity, altered mental status, fever, chills	Must remove pump and catheter; antibiotics per cultures
Postdural puncture headache	Fronto-occipital postural headache	Conservative management with rest and fluids; rarely epidural blood patch required if symptoms persist >2 wk
Pump malfunction (overinfusion)	Lower-than-expected reservoir volume at time of pump refill; intrathecal medication side effects, such as sedation, respiratory depression, lower extremity weakness, bradycardia, and so forth	Pump replacement
Pump malfunction (underinfusion)	Greater-than-expected reservoir volume at time of pump refill; diminishing analgesia; may provoke baclofen or clonidine withdrawal symptoms	Monitoring considered if underinfusion is mild and patient asymptomatic; may require pump replacement
Pump motor stall	Sudden loss of analgesia; may provoke life-threatening withdrawal syndrome with baclofen	Supportive care, pump replacement
Catheter malfunction	Decreased analgesia, inability to withdraw CSF from catheter access port, greater-than-expected reservoir volume at time of pump refill; may provoke baclofen or clonidine withdrawal symptoms; confirm with imaging	Intrathecal catheter revision (kinking of catheter) or replacement (catheter tip obstruction)
Catheter tip granuloma	Diminishing analgesia, new neurologic symptoms; associated with high doses and high concentrations of infusate	If no neurologic symptoms are present use less concentrated solution and monitor symptoms. The development of neurologic symptoms necessitates intrathecal catheter revision or replacement and myelopathy may require surgical decompression.

Abbreviations: CSF, cerebrospinal fluid; IV, intravenous.

as reduced systemic opioid use. Breakthrough pain management using patient-controlled intrathecal analgesia (PCIA) was also assessed, with PCIA showing higher efficacy (65% reduction in pain vs 47%) and faster median onset (10 minutes vs 30 minutes) as compared with traditional breakthrough analgesics.

- Cost-effectiveness: To address cost-effectiveness, a 2013 study showed that in patients with high-cost conventional medication regimens, IDD (including the cost of implantation) reached cost-effectiveness in an average of 7.4 months; 19% of these patients reached cost-effectiveness in less than 6 months.[16] In addition Deer and colleagues[8] reported that IDD using morphine or ziconotide reaches cost-effectiveness at 7 months and 10 months, respectively, as compared with a brand name oral regimen, even after accounting for the cost of implantation, pump refills, and pump reprogramming.

Intrathecal Drug Delivery and Ongoing Oncologic Care

Initiation and continuation of intrathecal therapy need not interfere with chemotherapy or radiotherapy regimens and in fact may allow patients to tolerate aggressive treatment more comfortably. Some chemotherapy protocols may require that IDDS implantation be timed to avoid a white cell count or platelet count nadir.

Radiation therapy does affect the battery life of IDDS and may in rare cases result in electrical failure. The pump may be protected by lead shielding and, if possible, through radiation field avoidance. If radiation is being performed for pain control, a temporary catheter may be used until this therapy becomes effective.

Patients with IDDS can safely undergo imaging studies such as radiographs, computed tomography (CT) scans, positron emission tomography (PET) scans, and nuclear medicine studies. However the function of the IDDS may be affected by magnetic resonance imaging (MRI) and manufacturer instructions should be consulted. In regards to the most commonly implanted IDDS, the SynchroMed II, exposure to the magnetic field may cause the pump rotor to pause during the scan.[17] In the authors' experience the pump motor resumes normal running conditions after the patient exits the magnetic field and the authors do not routinely interrogate the IDDS after MRI scans. A 2011 study showed "virtually no technical or medical complications" in 43 patients with the Synchromed II who received MRI scans over a 3-year period.[18]

VERTEBRAL AUGMENTATION

Osseous metastatic disease is common in patients with advanced cancer, and spine lesions are particularly common in patients with multiple myeloma as well as breast, prostate, renal cell, thyroid, and lung cancers. Spine lesions may lead to vertebral compression fractures (VCFs) that can cause debilitating pain and reduced function.

Although some patients improve with rest, analgesics, physical therapy, and bracing, pain can persist or be so severe that it compromises function. Open surgical repair carries risk of significant morbidity and is reserved for existing or impending myelopathy.

Vertebroplasty and kyphoplasty are minimally invasive procedures used to treat painful VCFs. Vertebroplasty aims to stabilize painful VCFs with injection of the bone cement polymethyl methacrylate (PMMA) into the vertebral body. Kyphoplasty differs in that the injection of PMMA is preceded by the inflation of a percutaneously placed intravertebral balloon to create a cavity, with or without attempted restoration of vertebral height (**Figs. 2** and **3**). There is controversy about the benefits of

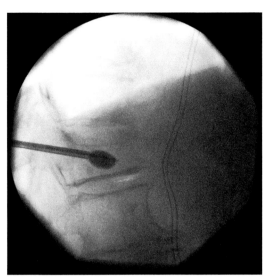

Fig. 2. Fluoroscopic lateral view of kyphoplasty with a trocar and balloon visible in the collapsed vertebral body.

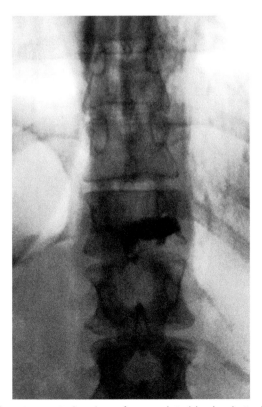

Fig. 3. Fluoroscopic anteroposterior view of a completed kyphoplasty showing cement in the vertebral body.

kyphoplasty over vertebroplasty, though the most recent data support the use of kyphoplasty in the cancer population.[19,20]

Indications

- Cancer-related acute or subacute (<6 months) painful pathologic VCF
- Moderate to severe axial spine pain at the levels of known VCFs
- Pain refractory to conservative treatment for at least 2 weeks

Contraindications

- Local or systemic infection
- Coagulopathy
- Allergy to contrast dye or polymethyl methacrylate
- Unfavorable fracture anatomy: severe vertebral body collapse, posterior vertebral body wall involvement, fragment retropulsion or tumor extension into the spinal canal, or severe spinal stenosis on computed tomography or MRI
- Radicular pain or radiculopathy (relative contraindication)
- Neurologic deficits (relative contraindication)

Complications

The most common complication is cement leakage into surrounding tissues. Although most of these cement extrusions are asymptomatic, they can rarely cause severe, life-threatening complications. Hematologic and infectious complications have also been reported[21] (**Table 3**).

Outcomes

Several studies and reviews on the use of vertebral augmentation for painful cancer-associated VCFs have been published in the last 10 years. These studies consistently demonstrate improvements in pain and function with a low incidence of adverse effects.[20,22]

- Berenson and colleagues[22] in 2011 published a randomized controlled trial of 134 patients with cancer comparing balloon kyphoplasty with nonsurgical treatment. Kyphoplasty was associated with improved pain scores at 1 week and 1 month, improved function, increased quality of life, reduced medication use, and markedly lower rates of bed rest. Adverse events were rare and nonserious.
- In 2011 the University of Texas MD Anderson Cancer Center reported their outcomes in 407 patients with 1156 VCFs who received vertebroplasty or kyphoplasty over a 7.5-year period. They reported reduced pain scores and reduced incidences of fatigue, depression, anxiety, and drowsiness following the procedure. Three serious complications, including 2 cases of symptomatic epidural extravasation requiring open surgery and one case of vertebral body infection, occurred in this series.[20]

NEUROLYTIC PLEXUS BLOCKS

Neurolysis of a sympathetic nervous system plexus, typically using dehydrated alcohol or phenol, is indicated for patients experiencing cancer-associated visceral pain. Pain relief typically lasts for months, and the procedure can be repeated if necessary. The celiac plexus, superior hypogastric plexus, and ganglion impar are the most common targets for the treatment of upper abdominal, pelvic, and perineal cancer pain, respectively. These procedures are summarized in **Table 4**.

Table 3
Complications of vertebral augmentation

Complication	Effect	Management
Cement extrusion into spinal canal	Transient or permanent paralysis, radiculopathy, or paresthesias	Emergent surgical decompression
Cement extrusion into neural foramen	Transient or permanent radiculopathy	Conservative management, rarely surgical intervention
Cement extrusion into intervertebral disk	Usually asymptomatic, rarely may result in scans diskitis	Conservative management, rarely surgical intervention
Cement embolus	Usually asymptomatic, rarely may result in symptomatic pulmonary embolus	Supportive management as indicated
Fat embolus	Varies; can be asymptomatic or cause transient hypotension, respiratory failure, or life-threatening cardiac collapse	Conservative management if minimally symptomatic, may require ACLS with serious emboli
Epidural hematoma	Transient or permanent paralysis	Emergent surgical decompression
Infection	Superficial skin infection, rarely epidural abscess, osteomyelitis, or diskitis	Oral or IV antibiotics as indicated, rarely surgical debridement
Allergic reaction	Anaphylaxis: associated with contrast dye and polymethyl methacrylate	Epinephrine, ACLS as needed
Rib fractures	Chest wall pain	Conservative management

Abbreviations: ACLS, advanced cardiac life support; IV, intravenous.

Table 4
Neurolytic plexus blocks

Procedure Location	Indications	Possible Adverse Effects
Celiac plexus	Upper abdominal visceral pain from malignant tumors of the pancreas, hepatobiliary system, small intestine, stomach, spleen, ascending colon, or adrenal glands	Transient hypotension Diarrhea Transient or permanent spinal cord damage (rare)
Superior hypogastric plexus	Visceral pelvic pain from malignant primary or metastatic tumor in the ovary, uterus, cervix, bladder, rectum, or prostate	Neuraxial injection Diskitis Bladder injury Intravascular injection Retroperitoneal hematoma
Ganglion impar	Perineal pain from rectal or anal cancers or metastatic perineal lesions	Rectal perforation Local infection Local bleeding Intravascular injection

Celiac Plexus Neurolysis

Neurolysis of the celiac plexus (NCPB) is the most common interventional procedure performed for cancer pain and is highly efficacious for upper abdominal visceral pain. It is commonly used in patients with pancreatic cancer, cholangiocarcinoma, and gastric cancer.

The celiac plexus is a network of sympathetic ganglia that transmits nociceptive signals from the pancreas, gallbladder, other hepatobiliary structures, distal stomach, small intestine, and large intestine as far distal as the transverse colon.

There are several approaches to the celiac plexus, the most common being a percutaneous bilateral retrocrural approach using fluoroscopy or CT guidance (**Figs. 4** and **5**). Patients are placed prone and the needles advanced under image guidance to the vicinity of the celiac plexus or the splanchnic nerves. Contrast media is injected to assure appropriate positioning. Local anesthetic is first injected followed by the neurolytic agent, typically 50% to 75% dehydrated alcohol.

Alternate methods for celiac plexus neurolysis are described, including a transesophageal endoscopic ultrasound-guided approach and an anterior transabdominal approach with CT or ultrasound guidance. Intraoperative blockade at the time of diagnostic or therapeutic laparotomy can be performed in order to denervate the celiac plexus under direct vision. There have not been any significant differences found among techniques in terms of efficacy or morbidity.[23]

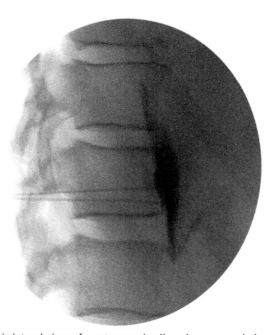

Fig. 4. Fluoroscopic lateral view of a retrocrural celiac plexus neurolysis.

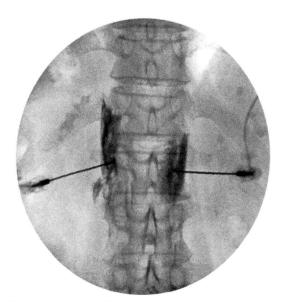

Fig. 5. Fluoroscopic anteroposterior view of a retrocrural celiac plexus neurolysis.

Indications

- Upper abdominal visceral pain
- Malignant primary or metastatic tumor in the pancreas, hepatobiliary system, stomach, spleen, small intestine, ascending colon cancer, or adrenal glands

Contraindications

- Local or systemic infection
- Coagulopathy
- Hemodynamic instability or hypovolemia
- Significant local anatomic abnormalities precluding safe needle placement

Complications

Neurolytic celiac plexus blockade is generally a safe and well-tolerated procedure. Rare but serious complications have been reported, including transient or permanent spinal cord damage and/or neurologic damage as a result of spread of the neurolytic agent to the neuraxial structures or damage to an anterior spinal artery. Serious complications are very rare, with an incidence of less than 0.2% in one series of 2730 neurolytic celiac plexus blocks.[24] Side effects are summarized in **Box 1**.

Box 1
Adverse effects associated with celiac plexus neurolysis

Transient hypotension due to splanchnic vasodilation

Diarrhea due to unopposed parasympathetic tone

Needle site pain

Transient or permanent spinal cord damage and paraplegia due to spread of the neurolytic agent to the nerve roots, epidural space, or intrathecal space

Neurologic dysfunction due to damage to an anterior spinal artery, such as the artery of Adamkiewicz, disrupting the vulnerable arterial supply of the spinal cord

---

Outcomes

Numerous case series, meta-analyses, and randomized controlled trials report favorable outcomes with celiac plexus neurolysis. Improvement in pain scores and reduced opioid consumption have been reported in most published reports, and some articles have demonstrated improved survival and quality of life.[23–28]

- The first large-scale meta-analysis was performed by Eisenberg and colleagues[29] in 1995 and described 1145 patients in 24 studies. They reported that 89% of patients archived good to excellent pain relief at 2 weeks, with partial to complete pain relief persisting at 3 months in 90% of patients. They also found a low rate of serious adverse events.
- A controlled trial by Wong and colleagues[25] published in 2004 randomly assigned 100 patients with unresectable pancreatic cancer with mild to moderate pain (visual analog scale 3/10 to 5/10) to either percutaneous NCPB or systemic analgesia therapy and a sham injection. At 1 week, pain and quality-of-life scores were improved with NCPB and improvement in pain lasted over time. Opioid consumption, opioid side effects, quality of life over time, and life expectancy were not different between groups. However, this study has been criticized for excluding patients with severe pain, in whom celiac plexus is most often performed and in whom improvements in quality of life, opioid consumption, and opioid side effects may be most pronounced.
- A large 2013 systematic review of celiac plexus neurolysis included 59 publications that used the percutaneous NCPB approach. Meta-analyses showed that NCPB improved pain, reduced opioid consumption, and reduced rates of side effects, including constipation, nausea, and vomiting, as compared with standard analgesic therapy.[23]
- A 2010 meta-analysis of the endoscopic approach for NCPB for pancreatic cancer included 5 studies totaling 119 patients and reported efficacy in alleviating abdominal pain in 73% of patients.[26]

Superior Hypogastric Plexus Neurolysis

The primary indication for superior hypogastric neurolytic block (SHNB) is visceral pelvic pain, most commonly from malignancy of the ovary, uterus, cervix, bladder,

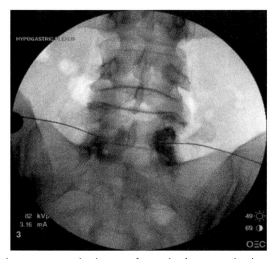

Fig. 6. Fluoroscopic anteroposterior image of superior hypogastric plexus neurolysis.

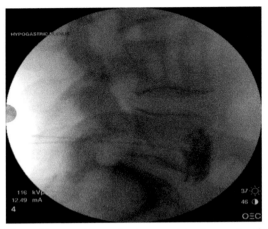

Fig. 7. Fluoroscopic lateral image of superior hypogastric plexus neurolysis.

rectum or prostate. The superior hypogastric plexus lies on the anterior surface of the L4 and L5 vertebral bodies and upper sacrum. A posterior percutaneous approach is used, though transdiscal, CT-guided, and ultrasound-guided approaches have been reported (**Figs. 6** and **7**).[30]

Indications

- Pelvic visceral pain secondary to malignant disease of the pelvic organs

Contraindications

- Local or systemic infection
- Coagulopathy
- Significant local anatomic abnormalities precluding safe needle placement

Complications
Reports in the literature of complications from SHNB are rare. Potential complications are summarized in **Box 2**.

Outcomes
The literature supporting SHNB is in the form of case reports, prospective case series, and one randomized controlled trial. These studies reliably demonstrate good to excellent pain relief for most patients and reduced opioid consumption without significant adverse effects.[31,32]

Box 2
Adverse effects associated with superior hypogastric plexus neurolysis
Neuraxial injection causing neurologic damage to the cauda equina
Diskitis
Bladder injury
Intravascular injection
Retroperitoneal hematoma

Ganglion Impar Neurolysis

The ganglion impar, also known as the ganglion of Walther, is a solitary ganglion located on the anterior surface of the sacrum. It provides nociceptive and sympathetic supply to perineum and neurolysis is indicated in refractory pain as a result of rectal, anal, vulvar, or other perineal cancers.

Neurolytic block of the ganglion impar is most commonly performed using a percutaneous transcoccygeal approach with fluoroscopic guidance (**Fig. 8**).[33] The anococcygeal approach has also been used, as have CT-guided approaches.[34]

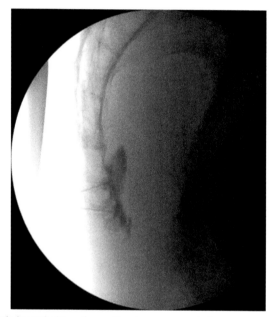

Fig. 8. Fluoroscopic lateral view of ganglion impar neurolysis.

Indications

- Perineal pain
- Malignant primary or metastatic lesion of the vulva, rectum, anus, or perineum

Contraindications

- Local or systemic infection
- Coagulopathy (relative contraindication)
- Significant local anatomic abnormalities precluding safe needle placement

Complications

Reports in the literature of complications are rare. Potential complications are summarized in **Box 3**.

Outcomes

Data regarding the efficacy of neurolytic ganglion impar block for cancer-associated perineal pain are limited to case reports and case series but consistently report improved pain with no significant adverse effects.[32–36]

| **Box 3** |
| **Adverse effects associated with ganglion impar neurolysis** |
| Rectal perforation |
| Local infection |
| Local bleeding |
| Intravascular injection |

Peripheral Nerve Neurolytic Blockade

There are growing reports of neurolysis of peripheral nerves for the management of intractable cancer pain localized to a specific nerve distribution. Phenol is the most commonly used neurolytic because of its comparatively high viscosity and tendency to remain in a localized area after injection as well as its intrinsic local anesthetic activity and lack of discomfort on injection. Peripheral neurolysis is largely restricted to nerves without significant motor activity, so function is minimally impaired following neurolysis. However, in end-of-life situations, or when tumor involvement has already compromised neural function, the benefit of improved pain control with neurolysis may outweigh the risk of lost motor function.

Intercostal Neurolysis

Intercostal neurolysis is indicated for somatic pain arising from metastatic disease to the ribs or chest wall. The intercostal neurovascular bundle runs along the inferior border of each rib and can be targeted percutaneously with ultrasound and/or fluoroscopy, though ultrasound is increasingly the preferred modality because of the ability to image, and avoid, the pleura. At a point 8 to 10 cm lateral to the midline a needle is inserted and advanced inferior to the rib, taking care to remain superficial to the pleura at all times. A diagnostic injection can be performed if desired, though the authors' favored approach is to proceed directly to neurolytic blockade with phenol (**Figs. 9** and **10**).

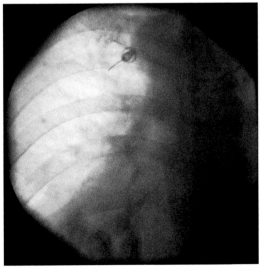

Fig. 9. Fluoroscopic view of intercostal neurolysis with the needle tip inferior to the rib.

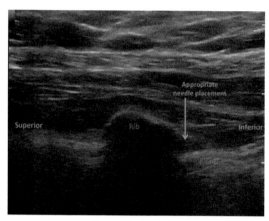

Fig. 10. Ultrasound view of intercostal neurolysis with appropriate needle position indicated.

Indications

- Somatic chest wall or rib pain
- Primary or metastatic lesion of the breast, lung, rib, or chest wall

Contraindications

- Local or systemic infection
- Coagulopathy
- Severe pulmonary disease requiring use of accessory muscles for ventilation (applicable if procedure is performed bilaterally and/or on multiple levels)

Complications

- Pneumothorax
- Hematoma
- Infection
- Intravascular injection
- Neuraxial spread
- Neuritis

Outcomes

Published reports are limited to case reports and case series.[37] The largest series to date published in 2007 describes 25 patients with metastatic rib lesions who underwent neurolytic intercostal block. This study found that 80% of the patients noted greater than 50% improvement in pain and 56% reduced their analgesic use after the procedure.[38]

Trigeminal Neurolysis

The trigeminal nerve is the fifth cranial nerve and is responsible for sensation over much of the face and motor function of the muscles of mastication. Trigeminal ganglion neurolysis is indicated for patients with head and neck cancer and somatic or neuropathic pain in the trigeminal distribution. Neurolysis will denervate the ipsilateral muscles of mastication, though this is typically not clinically significant so long as only unilateral blockade is performed.

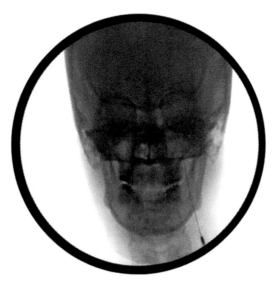

Fig. 11. Fluoroscopic anteroposterior view of trigeminal neurolysis with the needle placed within the foramen ovale.

Trigeminal neurolysis is technically challenging and should only be performed after specific training in the technique. The ganglion is accessed via the foramen ovale using fluoroscopic or CT guidance, typically followed by neurolysis with phenol or glycerol (**Figs. 11** and **12**).

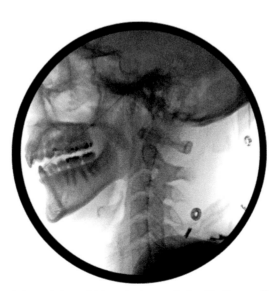

Fig. 12. Fluoroscopic lateral view of trigeminal neurolysis with the needle in an appropriate position within the foramen ovale.

Indications

- Neuropathic facial pain related to head and neck cancer

Contraindications

- Local or systemic infection
- Coagulopathy
- Tumor or severe anatomic distortion along the needle path

Complications

- Bleeding
- Dural puncture
- Intrathecal injection
- Intravascular injection
- Reactivation of herpes labialis or herpes zoster in the area
- Impaired corneal reflex and corneal anesthesia
- Neuritis

Outcomes

Most published reports on trigeminal neurolysis address its use for trigeminal neuralgia, with a reported success rate of 80% to 90% in these patients.[39] Although the literature for cancer pain is limited, given the high burden of pain in the head and neck cancer population, trigeminal neurolysis should be considered in these patients.[37]

Neurolytic Blocks of the Extremities

There have been several published reports of successful pain relief for extremity pain in patients with severe cancer pain at the end of life. Neuropathic upper extremity pain has been treated with neurolysis of the brachial plexus using both interscalene and infraclavicular approaches.[37] Groin and lower extremity pain have been effectively treated with transforaminal injection of phenol with no reported complications.[40]

IMAGE-GUIDED PERCUTANEOUS TUMOR ABLATION

Painful bony metastatic disease is common in patients with cancer. While external beam radiation therapy remains the mainstay of treatment, approximately 20% to 30% of patients do not respond to radiation. Recent advances have been made in treating this population using image-guided tumor ablation. This technique involves percutaneous placement of a needle into painful bone metastases followed by thermal destruction using radiofrequency ablation (RFA) or cryoablation.[41]

Radiofrequency Ablation

RFA uses transmission of a high-frequency, alternating current from the needle electrode to the surrounding tissues, resulting in heating of the tissues and cell necrosis. Advantages to RFA include immediate cell death and control of lesion size and temperature. The primary disadvantage of RFA is that the zone of ablation is not readily seen in real time with available imaging modalities. Tissue displacement and temperature monitoring adjacent to important structures are used to limit damage to surround structures.[41,42]

Cryoablation

Cryoablation uses specialized cryoprobes with rapid expansion of pressurized argon to produce rapid tissue cooling, reaching $-100°C$ within a few seconds. An ice ball is formed, which is then actively thawed by instilling pressurized helium gas into the cryoprobes. Although cryoablation is more costly and more time consuming as compared with RFA, it has the distinct advantages of being able to monitor the lesion size in real time and the ability to produce multiple ablations simultaneously.[41,43]

Indications

- Moderate to severe pain
- Pain located in 1 to 2 focal areas
- Areas of pain correlate with known sites of bony metastatic lesions
- Lesions amenable to ablative therapy: osteolytic or mixed osteolytic/osteoblastic

Contraindications

- Lesion location within 1 cm of the spinal cord, major motor nerve, brain, artery of Adamkiewicz, bowel, or bladder
- Widespread painful bony metastases
- Severe coagulopathy
- Local or systemic infection

Complications

Complications of image-guided tumor ablation occur primarily as a result of thermal damage to surrounding normal tissues.

- Spinal cord injury
- Bowel of bladder dysfunction
- Neuritis
- Loss of motor or sensory function in an area
- Damage to vascular structures
- Exacerbation of preexisting tumor-cutaneous fistulas
- Bone fracture with large ablation areas
- Infection
- Hematoma

Outcomes

Radiofrequency ablation Radiofrequency ablation is the most studied modality of image-guided tumor ablation and has been shown to be efficacious.

- In a 2006 study of 62 patients who failed conventional therapies, including radiation and chemotherapy, 95% of patients achieved lasting reductions in pain following RFA.[44]
- In 2010, Dupuy and colleagues[42] published a report on 55 patients who received RFA for single painful bone metastases. At 1 and 3 months patients reported reduced pain and improved mood.

Cryoablation Cryoablation is less studied than RFA, but case series and reports have established the efficacy of this procedure.

- In a 2006 study, 14 patients with painful bony metastatic lesions received cryoablation. Pain scores, pain interference, and opioid consumption were all reduced and no serious complications were observed.[44]
- In 2010, Thacker and colleagues[45] studied the immediate outcomes of patients who received either cryoablation (n = 36) or RFA (n = 22). Although both groups experienced reductions in pain after the procedure, cryoablation was associated with reduced analgesic use in the first 24 hours and a shorter hospital stay.

OTHER INTERVENTIONAL TREATMENTS OF CANCER PAIN
Spinal Cord Stimulation

Spinal cord stimulation (SCS) for cancer pain is limited to case reports and one case series but has been used successfully for multiple types and locations of pain. There are reports of treating pain directly resulting from anal cancer, metastatic colon cancer, testicular cancer, and angiosarcoma, as well as post-thoracotomy and chemotherapy-induced peripheral neuropathy pain.[46–50]

Until recently, the frequent need for MRI in oncology has limited the use of SCS. However there are now MRI-compatible devices available, which may expand its indications to selected refractory cancer pain conditions.

Intrathecal Neurolysis

Intrathecal neurolysis was initially described in 1931 and is effective for the treatment of somatic cancer pain. Intrathecal neurolysis uses hypobaric alcohol or hyperbaric phenol and skilled patient positioning to selectively achieve neurolysis at target nerve roots. However, its use is limited by significant morbidity, including bowel and/or bladder dysfunction, motor weakness, neuritis, and paresthesias.

Appropriate candidates are patients with end-stage cancer and severe, refractory pain, particularly in situations in which motor function, bowel control, and bladder function have already been lost.[37,51] However, with the advent of less invasive treatment options, few clinicians are comfortable performing this procedure.

Neurosurgical Procedures

Destructive neurosurgical procedures have a role in patients with cancer for whom medical management is not sufficient and less invasive interventional techniques are not available or not effective. A 2011 review found the best evidence for cordotomy, with most of the 47 published articles reporting excellent, lasting pain relief. Favorable outcomes with myelotomy, dorsal root entry zone lesion, and thalamotomy were also reported.[52] The primary barrier to obtaining neurosurgical pain procedures is the lack of neurosurgeons suitably trained in these techniques.

SUMMARY

Interventional treatments are indicated for the treatment of many different cancer pain syndromes. These approaches should be considered early in the treatment course and should complement pharmacologic and other symptom management techniques to improve patient comfort and function and permit full participation in the oncologic care plan. An understanding of proper patient selection, management of patient and referring physician expectations, knowledge of the procedural risks and benefits of each interventional procedure, and adequate postprocedural management are necessary for optimizing outcomes in these patients.

REFERENCES

1. Vainio A, Auvinen A. Prevalence of symptoms among patients with advanced cancer: an international collaborative study. Symptom Prevalence Group. J Pain Symptom Manage 1996;12(1):3–10.
2. WHO pain relief ladder for cancer pain relief. Available at: www.who.int/cancer/palliative/painladder/en/. Accessed September 5, 2015.
3. Vargas-Schaffer G. Is the WHO analgesic ladder still valid? Twenty-four years of experience. Can Fam Physician 2010;56(6):514–7.

4. Miguel R. Interventional treatment of cancer pain: the fourth step in the World Health Organization analgesic ladder? Cancer Control 2000;7(2):149–56.

5. Brogan S, Junkins S. Interventional therapies for the management of cancer pain. J Support Oncol 2010;8(2):52–9.

6. Fine PG, Brogan S. Interventional approaches to treating cancer pain. Am Soc Clin Oncol Educ Book 2009;583–8.

7. Stearns L, Boortz-Marx R, Du Pen S, et al. Intrathecal drug delivery for the management of cancer pain: a multidisciplinary consensus of best clinical practices. J Support Oncol 2005;3(6):399–408.

8. Deer TR, Smith HS, Burton AW, et al. Comprehensive consensus based guidelines on intrathecal drug delivery systems in the treatment of pain caused by cancer pain. Pain Physician 2011;14(3):E283–312.

9. Deer TR, Prager J, Levy R, et al. Polyanalgesic Consensus Conference 2012: Recommendations for the Management of Pain by Intrathecal (Intraspinal) Drug Delivery: Report of an Interdisciplinary Expert Panel Neuromodulation 2012;15(5):436–66.

10. Engle MP, Vinh BP, Harun N, et al. Infectious complications related to intrathecal drug delivery system and spinal cord stimulator system implantations at a comprehensive cancer pain center. Pain Physician 2013;16(3):251–7.

11. Follett K, Boortz-Marx RL, Drake JM, et al. Prevention and management of intrathecal drug delivery and spinal cord stimulation system infections. Anesthesiology 2004;100(6):1582–94.

12. Smith TJ, Staats PS, Deer T, et al. Randomized clinical trial of an implantable drug delivery system compared with comprehensive medical management for refractory cancer pain: impact on pain, drug-related toxicity, and survival. J Clin Oncol 2002;20(19):4040–9.

13. Smith TJ, Coyne PJ, Staats PS, et al. An implantable drug delivery system (IDDS) for refractory cancer pain provides sustained pain control, less drug-related toxicity, and possibly better survival compared with comprehensive medical management (CMM). Ann Oncol 2005;16(5):825–33.

14. Burton AW, Rajagopal A, Shah HN, et al. Epidural and intrathecal analgesia is effective in treating refractory cancer pain. Pain Med 2004;5(3):239–47.

15. Brogan SE, Winter NB, Okifuji A. Prospective observational study of patient-controlled intrathecal analgesia. Reg Anesth Pain Med 2015;40(4):369–75.

16. Brogan SE, Winter NB, Abiodun A, et al. A cost utilization analysis of intrathecal therapy for refractory cancer pain: identifying factors associated with cost benefit. Pain Med 2013;14(4):478–86.

17. Shellock FG, Crivelli R, Venugopalan R. Programmable infusion pump and catheter: evaluation using 3-tesla magnetic resonance. Magn Reson Imaging 2008; 11(3):163–70.

18. De Andres J, Villanueva V, Palmisani S, et al. The safety of magnetic resonance imaging in patients with programmable implanted intrathecal drug delivery systems: a 3-year prospective study. Anesth Analg 2011;112(5):1124–9.

19. Fourney DR, Schomer DF, Nader R, et al. Percutaneous vertebroplasty and kyphoplasty for painful vertebral body fractures in cancer patients. J Neurosurg 2003;98(1 Suppl):21–30.

20. Burton AW, Mendoza T, Gebhardt R, et al. Vertebral compression fracture treatment with vertebroplasty and kyphoplasty: experience in 407 patients with 1,156 fractures in a tertiary cancer center. Pain Med 2011;12(12):1750–7.

21. Nussbaum DA, Gailloud P, Murphy K. A review of complications associated with vertebroplasty and kyphoplasty as reported to the Food and Drug Administration medical device related web site. J Vasc Interv Radiol 2004;15(11):1185–92.

22. Berenson J, Pflugmacher R, Jarzem P, et al. Balloon kyphoplasty versus non-surgical fracture management for treatment of painful vertebral body compression fractures in patients with cancer: a multicentre, randomised controlled trial. Lancet Oncol 2011;12(3):225–35.

23. Nagels W, Pease N, Dobbels P. Celiac plexus neurolysis for abdominal cancer pain: a systematic review. Pain Med 2013;14:1140–63.

24. Davies DD. Incidence of major complications of neurolytic coeliac plexus block. J R Soc Med 1993;86(5):264–6.

25. Wong GY, Schroeder DR, Carns PE, et al. Effect of neurolytic celiac plexus block on pain relief, quality of life, and survival in patients with unresectable pancreatic cancer: a randomized controlled trial. JAMA 2004;291(9):1092–9.

26. Kaufman M, Singh G, Das S, et al. Efficacy of endoscopic ultrasound-guided celiac plexus block and celiac plexus neurolysis for managing abdominal pain associated with chronic pancreatitis and pancreatic cancer. J Clin Gastroenterol 2010;44(2):127–34.

27. Yan BM, Myers RP. Neurolytic celiac plexus block for pain control in unresectable pancreatic cancer. Am J Gastroenterol 2007;102(2):430–8.

28. Staats PS, Hekmat H, Sauter P, et al. The effects of alcohol celiac plexus block, pain, and mood on longevity in patients with unresectable pancreatic cancer: a double-blind, randomized, placebo-controlled study. Pain Med 2001;2(1):28–34.

29. Eisenberg E, Carr DB, Chalmers TC. Neurolytic celiac plexus block for treatment of cancer pain: a meta-analysis. Anesth Analg 1995;80(2):290–5.

30. Bosscher H. Blockade of the superior hypogastric plexus block for visceral pelvic pain. Pain Pract 2001;1(2):162–70.

31. Plancarte R, de Leon-Casasola O, El-Helaly M, et al. Neurolytic superior hypogastric plexus block for chronic pelvic pain associated with cancer. Reg Anesth Pain Med 1997;22(6):562–8.

32. Plancarte-Sánchez R, Guajardo-Rosas J, Guillen-Nuñez R. Superior hypogastric plexus block and ganglion impar (Walther). Tech Reg Anesth Pain Manag 2005; 9(2 SPEC ISS):86–90.

33. Eker HE, Cok OY, Kocum A, et al. Transsacrococcygeal approach to ganglion impar for pelvic cancer pain: a report of 3 cases. Reg Anesth Pain Med 2008; 33(4):381–2.

34. Agarwal-Kozlowski K, Lorke DE, Habermann CR, et al. CT-guided blocks and neuroablation of the ganglion impar (Walther) in perineal pain: anatomy, technique, safety, and efficacy. Clin J Pain 2009;25(7):570–6.

35. Day M. Sympathetic blocks: the evidence. Pain Pract 2008;8(2):98–109.

36. Toshniwal GR, Dureja GP, Prashanth SM. Transsacrococcygeal approach to ganglion impar block for management of chronic perineal pain: a prospective observational study. Pain Physician 2007;10(5):661–6.

37. Koyyalagunta D, Burton AW. The role of chemical neurolysis in cancer pain. Curr Pain Headache Rep 2010;14(4):261–7.

38. Wong FC, Lee TW, Yuen KK, et al. Intercostal nerve blockade for cancer pain: effectiveness and selection of patients. Hong Kong Med J 2007;13(4):266–70.

39. Day M. Neurolysis of the trigeminal and sphenopalatine ganglions. Pain Pract 2001;1(2):171–82.

40. Candido KD, Philip CN, Ghaly RF, et al. Transforaminal 5% phenol neurolysis for the treatment of intractable cancer pain. Anesth Analg 2010;110(1):216–9.

41. Callstrom MR, Charboneau JW. Image-guided palliation of painful metastases using percutaneous ablation. Tech Vasc Interv Radiol 2007;10(2):120–31.

42. Dupuy DE, Liu D, Hartfeil D, et al. Percutaneous radiofrequency ablation of painful osseous metastases: a multicenter American College of Radiology Imaging Network trial. Cancer 2010;116(4):989–97.

43. Callstrom MR, Dupuy DE, Solomon SB, et al. Percutaneous image-guided cryoablation of painful metastases involving bone: multicenter trial. Cancer 2013; 119(5):1033–41.

44. Callstrom M, Charboneau J, Goetz M, et al. Image-guided ablation of painful metastatic bone tumors: a new and effective approach to a difficult problem. Skeletal Radiol 2006;35:1–15.

45. Thacker PG, Callstrom MR, Curry TB, et al. Palliation of painful metastatic disease involving bone with imaging-guided treatment: comparison of patients' immediate response to radiofrequency ablation and cryoablation. Am J Roentgenol 2011;197(2):510–5.

46. Yakovlev AE, Ellias Y. Spinal cord stimulation as a treatment option for intractable neuropathic cancer pain. Clin Med Res 2008;6(3–4):103–6.

47. Yakovlev AE, Resch BE. Spinal cord stimulation for cancer-related low back pain. Am J Hosp Palliat Care 2012;29(2):93–7.

48. Nouri KH, Brish EL. Spinal cord stimulation for testicular pain. Pain Med 2011; 12(9):1435–8.

49. Yakovlev AE, Resch BE, Karasev S. Treatment of cancer-related chest wall pain using spinal cord stimulation. Am J Hosp Palliat Care 2010;27(8):552–6.

50. Cata JP, Cordella JV, Burton AW, et al. Spinal cord stimulation relieves chemotherapy-induced pain: a clinical case report. J Pain Symptom Manage 2004;27(1):72–8.

51. Candido K, Stevens RA. Intrathecal neurolytic blocks for the relief of cancer pain. Best Pract Res Clin Anaesthesiol 2003;17(3):407–28.

52. Raslan AM, Cetas JS, McCartney S, et al. Destructive procedures for control of cancer pain: the case for cordotomy. J Neurosurg 2011;114(1):155–70.

Chronic Pain and the Opioid Conundrum

Lynn R. Webster, MD

KEYWORDS

- Chronic pain • Opioid analgesics • Government • Policy • Practice guidelines

KEY POINTS

- Prescribed opioids for chronic noncancer pain pose risks for the individual and society in the form of diversion, misuse, abuse, addiction, and death.
- Evidence supporting long-term use of opioids for the treatment of chronic noncancer pain is sparse, but it does appear that some carefully selected patients may indeed benefit from this treatment.
- State regulatory bodies and other policymaking entities have instituted a number of efforts to halt nonmedical use (ie, abuse) of opioids, with attendant implications for clinical practice as well as patient access to pain treatment.
- A clear understanding is essential for prescribers of opioids of the rapidly evolving, regulatory and policymaking developments, as clinical practice must comply with federal and state law.

INTRODUCTION

The conundrum of opioid prescribing is usually understood to refer to the need to adequately control pain in patients who derive benefits from opioids, while, at the same time, working to prevent misuse, addiction, overdose deaths, and other associated risks and side effects.[1] The conundrum should not be construed to somehow weigh the lives lost to addiction or overdose against those lost to suicide due to uncontrolled pain, as neither category of loss is acceptable.

LESSONS LEARNED FROM HISTORY

The opioid conundrum has always reflected the tension inherent in public discussion of agents that provide relief of excruciating pain, some of which was formerly untreatable, and the fear that long-term harm may result to the user. As early as the seventeenth century, English doctor Thomas Sydenham called laudanum (a mixture containing opium) "the most valuable drug in the world"; however, his colleague John Jones

Scientific Affairs, PRA Health Sciences, 3838 South 700 East, Suite 202, Salt Lake City, UT 84106, USA
E-mail address: lrwebstermd@gmail.com

Anesthesiology Clin 34 (2016) 341–355
http://dx.doi.org/10.1016/j.anclin.2016.01.002
1932-2275/16/$ – see front matter © 2016 Elsevier Inc. All rights reserved.

anesthesiology.theclinics.com

declared that long-term use would cause "intolerable anxiety, and depression and a miserable death."[2] In recent years, public discussions of opioid use in clinical practice for chronic pain are often fraught with emotion, strong views, and barriers born of context, depending on the position of the commentator, whether pain physician, pain patient, addiction expert, law enforcement official, regulator, lawmaker, pharmaceutical industry representative, or other stakeholder.

One constant throughout history has been that many people with chronic pain are stigmatized, relegated to a frequently invisible class in society. With the advent of the work in the 1950s of John Bonica, MD, often referred to as "the father" of modern pain medicine, a philosophy arose to treat people with pain humanely and professionally, using multidisciplinary care to address the biopsychosocial components of the experience of pain.[3] Unfortunately, in the decades since, Bonica's vision has not achieved widespread adoption, as a pure bio-medical model became easier to apply clinically than individualized treatment and more readily supported by financial interests that include the optimization of insurance payer profits and minimization of costs, as well as pharmaceutical industry profits.[4]

A cultural shift to address uncontrolled chronic pain, beginning in the early 1990s, resulted in an increase in the quantity of opioids prescribed, driven at times by the mistaken belief that opioids administered clinically were without significant risk.[2,5] This change in practice was motivated by compelling evidence that pain in a medical setting often went unrelieved, a circumstance that contributed to uncontrolled pain becoming identified as a public health problem.[5,6] A movement to define failure to control pain as professional misconduct ensued,[6] and in 2010 the International Association for the Study of Pain adopted a declaration stating that access to pain management is a fundamental human right.[7]

With the dawn of the twenty-first century, the rise in opioid use to control chronic pain began to coincide with increases in harm associated with prescription opioids, including nonmedical use (ie, abuse) of opioids.[8] This contributed to a climate of fear among clinicians who treat pain, including the following[2,9]:

- Fear of contributing to nonmedical use, addiction, diversion, and overdose deaths;
- Fear of risk to the clinician's continued ability to practice medicine;
- Fear of contributing to uncontrolled pain because of reluctance to prescribe when indicated;
- Fear of actual or perceived failure to meet the standard of care, which, in turn, could lead to regulatory sanctions, such as suspension or revocation of the physician's license to practice medicine or suspension or revocation of the physician's federal controlled substances registration;
- Fear of actual or perceived recklessness in prescribing, which, in turn, could lead to criminal prosecution by federal or state authorities.

Brief Background on Chronic Pain

Chronic pain is precisely that: chronic. It is pain that lasts beyond the period expected for healing, generally defined as more than 3 months.[10] Pain may begin as a symptom; however, when it persists, changes in the structure and function of the central nervous system (CNS) occur, making pain itself a disease.[10]

The prevalence of chronic pain in America has not diminished and is expected to increase as the population ages, giving urgency to the call for more and better solutions.[11] More than 100 million Americans struggle with some level of chronic pain.[10] Contributing to treatment complexity, many people with chronic pain have multiple issues that include comorbid psychiatric conditions,[12,13] social pressures, isolation, and lack of community support. In addition, uncontrolled moderate-to-severe post-surgical pain is common, increasing health care costs, delaying recovery, and raising the risk for progression to chronic pain.[14]

Brief Background on Opioid-Related Death, Misuse, Abuse, Addiction

The wider availability of pharmaceuticals that has accompanied more liberal prescribing patterns has coincided with higher rates of overdose deaths, misuse, emergency department (ED) visits, and admissions for substance-abuse treatment involving opioids and other controlled substances. **Figs. 1** and **2** illustrate the rise in opioid-related deaths in the United States from 1999 to 2013,[15,16] and how the trend coincides with opioid sales.[15–17]

Further findings include the following:

- In 2013, 6.5 million Americans age 12 or older, representing 2.5% of the population, were current nonmedical users of prescription drugs, including opioids, stimulants, and benzodiazepines.[18]
- Of the 16,235 deaths involving opioids, 6973 involved benzodiazepines.[19] Indeed, most deaths involved more than one substance, with opioids and benzodiazepines a commonly seen combination.
- In 2011, ED visits involving prescription opioids reached 420,040, up 153% from 2004.[20] Similarly, ED visits involving benzodiazepines rose 124% over the same period and numbered 501,207 in 2011.
- Admissions for substance-abuse treatment involving opiates other than heroin (ie, principally prescription opioids) have grown, rising from 2% of admissions in 2002 to 10% by 2012.[21]
- The number of methadone deaths is disproportionate to the number of prescriptions written, as reported by the Centers for Disease Control and Prevention:

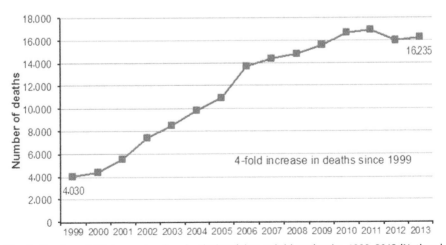

Fig. 1. Number of US drug poisoning deaths involving opioid analgesics, 1999–2013 (National Vital Statistics System Mortality Data). Drug poisoning deaths are identified using the *International Classification of Diseases, Tenth Revision* underlying cause of death codes X40–X44, X60–X64, X85, and Y10–Y14. Drug poisoning deaths involving opioid analgesics are the subset of drug poisoning deaths with a multiple cause of death code of T40.2–T40.4. (*Data from* Refs.[15,16])

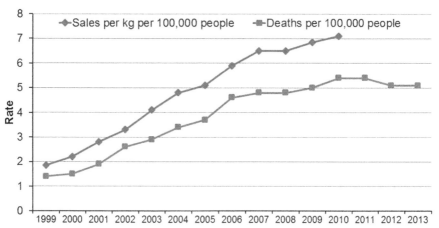

Fig. 2. Rates of prescription opioid sales and deaths, 1999–2013 (National Vital Statistics System; automation of reports and consolidated orders system of the Drug Enforcement Administration). (*Data from* Refs.[15–17])

methadone accounts for approximately 2% of opioid prescriptions written but is associated with one-third of deaths.[22] In 2009, 6 times as many people died of methadone-related overdose as a decade before.[22]

OPIOID EFFECTIVENESS DATA

A 2015 systematic review performed for a National Institutes of Health workshop to evaluate the evidence on opioids for chronic pain found the following[23]:

- Insufficient evidence to determine the effectiveness of long-term opioid therapy for improving chronic pain and function;
- A dose-dependent risk for serious harms, such as abuse, addiction, overdose, fractures, and cardiovascular events;
- Inadequate data to identify the medical conditions in patients for whom opioid use is most appropriate;
- Inadequate data to identify optimal regimens;
- Inadequate data to identify the treatment alternatives for those who are unlikely to benefit from opioids.

The following findings are from a review of more than 70 randomized trials that evaluated the benefits and harms of opioids for chronic noncancer pain[24]:

- Nearly all were short-term efficacy studies, lasting 16 weeks or less;
- Only 3 studies followed patients for longer than 4 months;
- Most studies excluded patients at high risk for substance abuse or with significant medical or psychiatric comorbidities.

The lack of long-term studies is frequently held up as evidence that no benefit has been demonstrated; however, this conclusion would overstate what the evidence allows. There are some studies (**Table 1**),[25–40] as well as clinical experience, that suggest that some patients do well long-term. Despite limitations that include open-label design, differing methodologies and inclusion/exclusion criteria and lack of nonopioid comparison groups, the studies in **Table 1** counter the argument that no evidence of

Table 1
Studies beyond 90 days of opioid effectiveness for chronic pain

Study, Year	Study Type	Maximum Observation Duration, mo	No. Evaluable
Noble et al,[25] 2008	Systematic review, meta-analysis	24	3079
Portenoy et al,[26] 2007	Prospective registry	36	219
Caldwell et al,[27] 2002	Open-label extension	7.5	295
Roth et al,[28] 2000	Open-label extension	6	58
		12	41
		18	15
Rauck et al,[29] 2008	Open-label, nonrandomized	6	126
McIlwain & Andieh,[30] 2005	Open-label extension	12	153
Wild et al,[31] 2010	Open-label, randomized, phase 3	12	1117
Allan et al,[32] 2005	Open-label, randomized, parallel group,	13	680
Bettoni,[33] 2006	Prospective, nonrandomized	24	14
Collado & Torres,[34] 2008	Prospective, nonrandomized	6	215
Fredheim et al,[35] 2006	Open-label, prospective, nonrandomized	9	12
Milligan et al,[36] 2001	Open-label, prospective, nonrandomized	12	532
Mystakidou et al,[37] 2003	Open-label, prospective, nonrandomized	10	529
Breivik et al,[38] 2010	Randomized, double-blind, placebo-controlled	6	199
Wen et al,[39] 2010	Open-label, extension	3	1127
		6	728
		12	154
Richarz et al,[40] 2013	Open-label, extension	12	112

Data from Refs.[25–40]

long-term benefit exists. Furthermore, the ethical difficulty of administering placebo to people with severe pain for prolonged periods of time precludes long-term double-blind, placebo-controlled studies.

Some additional findings illuminate several points for discussion, as follows:

- Many patients discontinue opioids because of inadequate analgesia or side effects[25];
- Opioids continue to demonstrate benefits for some patients who are able to continue treatment for at least 6 months[25];
- There is significant confounding of effectiveness by the high prevalence of psychiatric comorbidities in the population of opioid-treated patients[41];
- Noncompliance with opioid therapy increases with mental health issues.[42]

These findings must be factored into the discussion, while, at the same time, recognition is necessary that not all patients are likely to benefit with long-term opioid therapy and that the accompanying risks are significant.

ABUSE-DETERRENT TECHNOLOGY

Abuse-deterrent technologies in opioid formulations developed by the pharmaceutical industry have begun to demonstrate effectiveness in deterring nonmedical use, although results show lack of complete protection.[43–45] Studies of the reformulated oxycodone hydrochloride (HCl) extended-release (ER) tablets (Purdue Pharma LP, Stamford, CT), available since 2010, showed a decrease in preference by opioid-dependent subjects for oxycodone HCl ER as a primary drug of abuse, as well as reductions in diversion and poison center exposures after introduction of the reformulated product.[43–45] The largest drop was seen in nonoral routes of abuse, which decreased by 66%.[43] These results may not translate to less overall opioid abuse in the population, particularly if non–abuse-deterrent formulations remain available and are preferred by third-party payers as affordable pain treatment options.

THE PROBLEM WITH PAYER POLICIES

The health insurance system in the United States exacerbates the problem of suboptimal pain management. Lack of willingness by third-party payers to cover coordinated interdisciplinary care programs and certain nonmedication therapies (eg, physical therapy, psychotherapeutic modalities, complementary and alternative medicine approaches) as well as payer restrictions that limit the use of more expensive nonopioid analgesic medications often leave patients to suffer or drive them toward less effective treatments and drug therapies (both licit and illicit) with accompanying risk for a substance-use disorder.[4] Interdisciplinary care delivered in the context of a biopsychosocial model has a strong evidence base for efficacy and cost-effectiveness.[46] Unfortunately, access to interdisciplinary care is decreasing in the United States, even while access is increasing in other industrialized nations.[46] The number of US interdisciplinary pain care programs dropped from more than 1000 in 1999 to approximately 150 as of 2011, with roughly one available interdisciplinary program for every 670,000 sufferers of chronic pain.[46] An overhaul of the payer system would be necessary to require adequate coverage for evidence-based alternatives to opioids for chronic pain.

OPIOID RESEARCH STILL NEEDED

Given the crisis of unmet need for pain control, the question grows in importance of why the dearth of research and investment into effective and safer analgesic therapies is allowed to continue. At minimum, the following research questions pursuant to opioids and pain deserve greater focus:

- How does the individual patient's genome contribute to pain processing and opioid responsiveness?
- Why do different patients vary in response to different opioid molecules?
- How may a risk-benefit ratio be determined before, not after, opioids are prescribed?
- Is dose alone responsible for greater opioid-related harm, or do higher doses prescribed in patients with high pain intensity and more comorbidities lead to poorer outcomes?
- Which alternatives to opioids are safe and effective (eg, abuse-deterrent opioid formulations, cannabinoids, psychological and behavioral therapies, complementary and integrative therapies, such as mindfulness)?
- Were some opioid-related, overdose deaths that were attributed to unintentionality actually intentional to escape unrelenting physical pain or emotional misery from a multitude of psychological, social, and spiritual deficits?

REGULATORY CONSIDERATIONS

Efforts directed toward minimizing misuse, abuse, addiction, overdose mortality, and other harms associated with opioid use have included initiatives directed at limiting opioid dose and treatment duration.[47] However, severe chronic pain is not a short-term problem. Policy proposals aimed at decreasing harm are not feasible or humane if they skirt this reality.

Upper Dose Limits: Washington State

A guideline first published in 2007 by the Washington State Agency Medical Directors Group (AMDG) stated the following[48]:

- Doses higher than 120-mg oral morphine equivalents per day should rarely be given and "only after pain management consultation."

Elements from the guideline were passed into state law and began to be enforced in 2012. In addition to the dose limit that triggered expert consultation, the bill required close monitoring of patient outcomes.

Problems raised with this dose limit included the following[47,49]:

- Pain specialists for consultation were in short supply;
- The 120-mg ceiling guideline was reached without sufficient scientific support;
- The guideline specified a diagnosis of "noncancer" pain, setting up possible discrimination;
- Potential risk of false security in believing doses less than 120 mg are always "safe";
- Failure to emphasize the danger of cointoxication with benzodiazepines and other CNS depressants;
- Insufficient attention to harm-contributing factors, such as nonmedical opioid use, drug formulation impact, patient mental health and nonadherence, prescriber error, suicide, polysubstance use, and variable individual pharmacokinetics;
- Failure to address the increased risk of harm unique to the use of methadone to treat noncancer pain;
- Potential to worsen patient access to care, especially if the guideline were to become interpreted to be a "standard of care" and embraced more broadly (eg, other states, nationally).

An update to the AMDG guideline, issued in 2015, retained the 120-mg "yellow flag," citing evidence to support it, but also put new emphasis on the need for caution at any dose.[50]

Risk Evaluation and Mitigation Strategy Programs

The Food and Drug Administration (FDA) approved a risk evaluation and mitigation strategy (REMS) for ER and long-acting (LA) opioids to ensure benefits outweigh risks.[51] Manufacturers of opioids are now required to distribute medication guides and to provide prescribers with education programs, created through accredited continuing education providers and based on an FDA Blueprint. Prescribing clinicians are strongly encouraged to complete a REMS education program. Although the FDA action did not cover immediate-release formulations, prescribing clinicians should take equal care to assess risk and provide optimal follow-up and monitoring for patients on any controlled substances prescribed during the course of pain management.

Food and Drug Administration Labeling Changes

In response to requests to make labeling changes for opioid analgesics, the FDA enacted the following labeling changes for ER/LA opioids[52]:

- Emphasized the need to individualize treatment;
- Stated the pain must be severe *enough* to indicate treatment with ER/LA opioids;
- Recommended use only when alternatives are determined to be inadequate;
- Urged caution regarding coadministration with alcohol and with centrally-acting sedating medications;
- Placed firmer focus on assessment of patient daily activities and quality of life rather than pain scale alone;
- Urged caution regarding opioid use during pregnancy, including the risk of newborn infants experiencing neonatal abstinence syndrome when the mother consumed chronic opioids during pregnancy;
- Required studies beyond 12 weeks to assess risks of misuse, abuse, hyperalgesia, and addiction.

Rescheduling of Hydrocodone

On October 6, 2014, the Drug Enforcement Administration (DEA) moved hydrocodone from Schedule III to the more strictly regulated Schedule II, triggering the following changes[53]:

- Prescriptions became limited to no more than a 30-day supply;
- Patients must see doctors for each new refill;
- Prescriptions can no longer be phoned or faxed in.

The DEA cited growing problems with opioid-related abuse, addiction, and overdose deaths as the reason for stricter regulatory action.

In response to early indications that the regulation may be affecting patient access to pain medications, an Internet survey was conducted to gather information on the first 100 days of hydrocodone rescheduling. Administered through the National Fibromyalgia & Chronic Pain Association, the survey found that two-thirds of participants reported trouble filling prescriptions for hydrocodone combination products, and 15% reported negative impacts on physician-patient relationships.[54] The survey had 3000 participants, many with multiple pain diagnoses that included fibromyalgia (91%), low back pain (62%), and neck pain (44%).

PRINCIPLES OF PRACTICE

Opioids are imperfect but may be necessary even longterm for some patients. Patients being considered for chronic opioid therapy must be carefully evaluated, stratified by risk for problematic opioid usage, and monitored for therapeutic effects, adverse events, aberrant drug-related behaviors, and progress toward treatment goals. Practice guidelines are available, and all state, federal, and local controlled substances law must be followed. Regardless, pain is still a subjective experience and one that requires considerable clinical experience, judgment, and resources to treat effectively.

Opioid Guidelines from Professional Medical Societies

Several opioid-prescribing guidelines are available to assist clinicians. A published systematic review of 13 such guidelines gave high ratings to 2 publications[55]: the joint guideline of the American Pain Society (APS) and American Academy of Pain Medicine (AAPM)[56] and the guideline from the Canadian National Opioid Use Guideline

Table 2 Screening tools to assess patient risk before prescribing opioids		
Tool	**No. of Items**	**Method of Administration**
Opioid Risk Tool	5	Patient
Screener and Opioid Assessment for Patients with Pain	24, 14, or 5	Patient
Diagnosis, Intractability, Risk, and Efficacy Score	7	Clinician

Data from Refs.[56,59–62]

Group.[57,58] An expert panel took more than a year and reviewed 8000 studies to produce the joint APS/AAPM guideline.[56] Seven other guidelines were found to be of intermediate quality, and 4 guidelines were not recommended for use.

Guidelines found common ground in several areas, including recommending that prescribers of opioids do the following[55–58]:

- Obtain a detailed history and physical examination;
- Assess for abuse and addiction, perhaps using an opioid-specific tool[56,59–62](**Table 2**);
- Initiate an individual trial and titration regimen;
- Periodically reassess the patient for function, progress toward treatment goals, adverse events, and adherence to medical direction; see **Table 3** for suggested clinical monitoring tools[63,64];
- Possess special knowledge to prescribe methadone;
- Recognize risks of fentanyl patches;
- Titrate cautiously;
- Reduce doses by ≥25% to 50% when rotating to a different opioid;
- Use opioid risk assessment tools;
- Use written treatment agreements;
- Use urine drug testing to check for patient adherence;
- Check the state prescription drug monitoring database where available;
- Treat high-risk patients with more frequent and stringent monitoring and comanagement with mental health and addiction specialists;
- Consider reasons for repeated escalations in opioid dose;
- Consider opioid rotation with adverse effects or ineffective analgesia;
- Discontinue opioid therapy through tapering when repeated aberrant drug-related behaviors are observed.

These principles of practice coincide with state practice requirements, which are frequently listed on the Web site of each state's medical board or professional licensing agency. Many states have adopted standards set by the Federation of State Medical Boards (FSMB), which has issued and updated a Model Policy[65] (**Box 1**).

Table 3 Monitoring tools after initiation of opioid therapy		
Tool	**No. of Items**	**Method of Administration**
Pain Assessment and Documentation Tool	41	Clinician
Current Opioid Misuse Measure	17	Patient

Data from Refs.[63,64]

Box 1
FSMB model policy for the use of opioid analgesics in the treatment of chronic pain

1. Thorough evaluation and risk stratification with an indication for prescribed opioids supported by history, physical, and appropriate tests before prescribing

2. Written treatment plan with stated objectives and consideration of pharmacologic and nonpharmacologic treatment modalities as appropriate

3. Informed consent on risks/benefits and an agreement for treatment outlining physician/patient responsibilities

4. Opioid trial following consideration of safer alternatives at lowest possible dose, titrated to effect

5. Regular review of the course of treatment to evaluate progress toward treatment objectives and to monitor adherence with medical direction, adjusting treatment when necessary, using "5 A's": analgesia, activity, adverse effects, aberrant substance-related behaviors, and affect

6. Periodic drug testing to ensure patient adherence (eg, urine testing, pill counts, prescription database checks)

7. Referrals for additional and specialist evaluation and treatment if necessary

8. Continually weigh benefits versus risk of opioid therapy and institute opioid discontinuation plan if necessary (eg, resolution of pain, intolerable side effects, inadequate analgesia, significant aberrant use, deteriorating function)

9. Accurate and complete records that include documentation of all of the above and all prescription orders

10. Familiarity and compliance with all state and federal laws and regulations regarding controlled substances

Abbreviation: FSMB, Federation of State Medical Boards.
  Data from Ref.[65]

Health Care Providers Are Not Alone

Co-occurrence of mental health disorders with chronic pain places patients at higher risk for misuse, drug-drug interactions, and overdose.

Consultation should be considered when health care providers feel that the patient may benefit from other resources.[56] Keep in mind there is an approximately 50% overlap of pain disorders with psychiatric disorders.[66–69] Furthermore, there is an approximately 60% overlap of psychiatric disorders with addiction disorders.[70]

For long-term pain management, opioids are only one tool; interdisciplinary and multimodal care are optimal.[71] Patients may not benefit from opioids as follows:[71]

- Opioids appear to be causing significant side effects;
- Opioids do not seem to be effectively leading to attainment of specified goals;
- Patients gain analgesia from opioid therapy but are at risk of misuse or overuse.

SUMMARY

- Opioids are an imperfect option for all pain states but the only treatment that works for many pain conditions;
- Whenever possible, an equally efficacious nonopioid therapy should be offered, even if the cost is greater;
- When initiating opioid therapy, risk assessment leading to risk stratification should be implemented;

- To support optimal clinical decisions regarding treatment choices, significant change is necessary to the payer system;
- Familiarity with opioid practice guidelines, regulatory requirements, and laws pertaining to controlled substances is an obligation of all prescribers.

ACKNOWLEDGMENTS

Beth Dove of Dove Medical Communications, LLC, Salt Lake City, Utah, provided medical writing for this article.

REFERENCES

1. Ballantyne JC. Opioid analgesia: perspectives on right use and utility. Pain Physician 2007;10:479–91.
2. Rhodin A. The rise of opiophobia: is history a barrier to prescribing? J Pain Palliat Care Pharmacother 2006;20:31–2.
3. Bonica JJ. The management of pain, with special emphasis on the use of block in diagnosis, prognosis and therapy. Philadelphia: Lea & Febiger; 1953.
4. Schatman ME, Webster LR. The health insurance industry: perpetuating the opioid crisis through policies of cost-containment and profitability. J Pain Res 2015;8:153–8.
5. Bennett DS, Carr DB. Opiophobia as a barrier to the treatment of pain. J Pain Palliat Care Pharmacother 2002;16:105–9.
6. Brennan F, Carr DB, Cousins MJ. Pain management: a fundamental human right. Anesth Analg 2007;105:205–21.
7. International Pain Summit of the International Association for the Study of Pain. Declaration of Montréal: declaration that access to pain management is a fundamental human right. J Pain Palliat Care Pharmacother 2011;25:29–31.
8. Gilson AM, Ryan KM, Joranson DE, et al. A reassessment of trends in the medical use and abuse of opioid analgesics and implications for diversion control: 1997-2002. J Pain Symptom Manage 2004;28:176–88.
9. Webster LR, Dove B. Avoiding opioid abuse while managing pain: a guide for practitioners. North Branch (MN): Sunrise River Press; 2007.
10. Institute of Medicine (US) Committee on Advancing Pain Research, Care, and Education. Relieving pain in America: a blueprint for transforming prevention, care, education, and research. Washington, DC: National Academies Press (US); 2011.
11. Woolf AD, Pfleger B. Burden of major musculoskeletal conditions. Bull World Health Organ 2003;81:646–56.
12. Tsang A, Von Korff M, Lee S, et al. Common chronic pain conditions in developed and developing countries: gender and age differences and comorbidity with depression-anxiety disorders. J Pain 2008;9:883–91.
13. Ohayon MM, Schatzberg AF. Chronic pain and major depressive disorder in the general population. J Psychiatr Res 2010;44:454–61.
14. McGrath B, Elgendy H, Chung F, et al. Thirty percent of patients have moderate to severe pain 24 hr after ambulatory surgery: a survey of 5,703 patients. Can J Anaesth 2004;51:886–91.
15. Chen LH, Hedegaard H, Warner M. QuickStats: rates of deaths from drug poisoning and drug poisoning involving opioid analgesics—United States, 1999–2013. MMWR Morb Mortal Wkly Rep 2015;64:32.

16. Warner M, Chen LH, Hedegaard H, et al. Trends in drug-poisoning deaths involving opioid analgesics and heroin: United States, 1999-2012. CDC Health E-Stats; 2014.

17. Centers for Disease Control and Prevention. CDC vital signs: prescription painkiller overdoses in the US. 2011. Available at: http://www.cdc.gov/vitalsigns/painkilleroverdoses/. Accessed October 29, 2015.

18. Substance Abuse and Mental Health Services Administration. Results from the 2013 national survey on drug use and health: summary of national findings. Rockville (MD): Substance Abuse and Mental Health Services Administration; 2014. NSDUH Series H-48, HHS Publication No. (SMA) 14–4863.

19. Centers for Disease Control and Prevention. Prescription drug overdose data: deaths from prescription overdose data (2013). Available at: http://www.cdc.gov/drugoverdose/data/overdose.html. Accessed September 23, 2015.

20. Substance Abuse and Mental Health Services Administration, Center for Behavioral Health Statistics and Quality, Center for Behavioral Health Statistics and Quality. The DAWN report: highlights of the 2011 drug abuse warning network (DAWN) findings on drug-related emergency department visits. Rockville (MD): Westat; 2013.

21. Substance Abuse and Mental Health Services Administration, Center for Behavioral Health Statistics and Quality. Treatment episode data set (TEDS): 2002-2012. National admissions to substance abuse treatment services. Rockville (MD): Substance Abuse and Mental Health Services Administration; 2014. BHSIS Series S-71, HHS Publication No. (SMA) 14-4850.

22. Centers for Disease Control and Prevention (CDC). Vital signs: prescription painkiller overdoses: use and abuse of methadone as a painkiller. 2012. Available at: http://www.cdc.gov/vitalsigns/MethadoneOverdoses. Accessed October 13, 2015.

23. Chou R, Turner JA, Devine EB, et al. The effectiveness and risks of long-term opioid therapy for chronic pain: a systematic review for a National Institutes of Health Pathways to Prevention Workshop. Ann Intern Med 2015;162(4):276–86.

24. Chou R, Ballantyne JC, Fanciullo GJ, et al. Research gaps on use of opioids for chronic noncancer pain: findings from a review of the evidence for an American Pain Society and American Academy of Pain Medicine clinical practice guideline. J Pain 2009;10:147–59.

25. Noble M, Tregear SJ, Treadwell JR, et al. Long-term opioid therapy for chronic noncancer pain: a systematic review and meta-analysis of efficacy and safety. J Pain Symptom Manage 2008;35:214–28.

26. Portenoy RK, Farrar JT, Backonja MM, et al. Long-term use of controlled-release oxycodone for noncancer pain: results of a 3-year registry study. Clin J Pain 2007;23:287–99.

27. Caldwell JR, Rapoport RJ, Davis JC, et al. Efficacy and safety of a once-daily morphine formulation in chronic, moderate-to-severe osteoarthritis pain: results from a randomized, placebo-controlled, double-blind trial and an open-label extension trial. J Pain Symptom Manage 2002;23:278–91.

28. Roth SH, Fleischmann RM, Burch FX, et al. Around-the-clock, controlled-release oxycodone therapy for osteoarthritis-related pain: placebo-controlled trial and long-term evaluation. Arch Intern Med 2000;160:853–60.

29. Rauck R, Ma T, Kerwin R, et al. Titration with oxymorphone extended release to achieve effective long-term pain relief and improve tolerability in opioid-naive patients with moderate to severe pain. Pain Med 2008;9:777–85.

30. McIlwain H, Ahdieh H. Safety, tolerability, and effectiveness of oxymorphone extended release for moderate to severe osteoarthritis pain: a one-year study. Am J Ther 2005;12:106–12.

31. Wild JE, Grond S, Kuperwasser B, et al. Long-term safety and tolerability of tapentadol extended release for the management of chronic low back pain or osteoarthritis pain. Pain Pract 2010;10:416–27.

32. Allan L, Richarz U, Simpson K, et al. Transdermal fentanyl versus sustained release oral morphine in strong-opioid naive patients with chronic low back pain. Spine 2005;30:2484–90.

33. Bettoni L. Transdermal fentanyl in rheumatology: two years' efficacy and safety in the treatment of chronic pain. [Fentanyl transdermico in reumatologia: efficacia e sicurezza a due anni nel trattamento del dolore cronico]. Recenti Prog Med 2006; 97:308–10.

34. Collado F, Torres LM. Association of transdermal fentanyl and oral transmucosal fentanyl citrate in the treatment of opioid naive patients with severe chronic noncancer pain. J Opioid Manag 2008;4:111–5.

35. Fredheim OM, Kaasa S, Dale O, et al. Opioid switching from oral slow release morphine to oral methadone may improve pain control in chronic non-malignant pain: a nine-month follow-up study. Palliat Med 2006;20:35–41.

36. Milligan K, Lanteri-Minet M, Borchert K, et al. Evaluation of long-term efficacy and safety of transdermal fentanyl in the treatment of chronic noncancer pain. J Pain 2001;2:197–204.

37. Mystakidou K, Parpa E, Tsilika E, et al. Long-term management of noncancer pain with transdermal therapeutic system-fentanyl. Pain 2003;4:298–306.

38. Breivik H, Ljosaa TM, Stengaard-Pedersen K, et al. A 6-month, randomized, placebo- controlled evaluation of efficacy and tolerability of a low-dose 7-day buprenorphine transdermal patch in osteoarthritis patients naive to potent opioids. Scand J Pain 2010;1:122–41.

39. Wen W, Munera CL, Dain B, et al. Long-term use of buprenorphine transdermal system (BTDS) in patients with chronic pain. Poster Presented at Pain Week. Las Vegas (NV), September 8–11, 2010.

40. Richarz U, Waechter S, Sabatowski R, et al. Sustained safety and efficacy of once-daily hydromorphone extended-release (OROS® hydromorphone ER) compared with twice-daily oxycodone controlled-release over 52 weeks in patients with moderate to severe chronic noncancer pain. Pain Pract 2013;13:30–40.

41. Sullivan MD, Edlund MJ, Zhang L, et al. Association between mental health disorders, problem drug use, and regular prescription opioid use. Arch Intern Med 2006;166:2087–93.

42. Wasan AD, Butler SF, Budman SH, et al. Psychiatric history and psychologic adjustment as risk factors for aberrant drug-related behavior among patients with chronic pain. Clin J Pain 2007;23:307–15.

43. Butler SF, Cassidy TA, Chilcoat H, et al. Abuse rates and routes of administration of reformulated extended-release oxycodone: initial findings from a sentinel surveillance sample of individuals assessed for substance abuse treatment. J Pain 2013;14:351–8.

44. Severtson SG, Bartelson BB, Davis JM, et al. Reduced abuse, therapeutic errors, and diversion following reformulation of extended-release oxycodone in 2010. J Pain 2013;14:1122–30.

45. Cicero TJ, Ellis MS, Surratt HL. Effect of abuse-deterrent formulation of OxyContin. N Engl J Med 2012;367:187–9.

46. Schatman ME. Interdisciplinary chronic pain management: international perspectives. Pain: Clin Updates 2012;20:1–5. Available at: http://www.iasp-pain.org/PublicationsNews/NewsletterIssue.aspx?ItemNumber=2065.
47. Ziegler SJ. The proliferation of dosage thresholds in opioid prescribing policies and their potential to increase pain and opioid-related mortality. Pain Med 2015;16(10):1851–6.
48. Interagency guideline on opioid dosing for chronic non-cancer pain: an educational pilot to improve care and safety with opioid treatment. Olympia (WA): Washington State Agency Medical Directors' Group; 2007. Available at: http://www.agencymeddirectors.wa.gov/Files/2015AMDGOpioidGuideline.pdf.
49. Fishman SM, Webster LR. Unintended harm from opioid prescribing guidelines. Pain Med 2009;10:285–6.
50. Interagency guideline on prescribing opioids for pain. 3rd edition. Olympia (WA): Washington State Agency Medical Directors' Group; 2015. Available at: http://www.agencymeddirectors.wa.gov/Files/2015AMDGOpioidGuideline.pdf.
51. U.S. Department of Health and Human Services, Food and Drug Administration. Risk evaluation and mitigation strategy (REMS) for extended-release and long-acting opioids. 2012. Available at: http://www.fda.gov/Drugs/DrugSafety/InformationbyDrugClass/ucm163647.htm. Accessed July 7, 2015.
52. U.S. Department of Health and Human Services, Food and Drug Administration. New safety measures announced for extended-release and long-acting opioids. 2013. Available at: http://www.fda.gov/Drugs/DrugSafety/InformationbyDrugClass/ucm363722.htm. Accessed October 29, 2015.
53. Drug Enforcement Administration, Department of Justice. Schedules of controlled substances: rescheduling of hydrocodone combination products from schedule III to schedule II. Final rule. Fed Regist 2014;79(163):49661–82. Available at: http://www.gpo.gov/fdsys/pkg/FR-2014-08-22/pdf/2014-19922.pdf. Accessed October 15, 2015.
54. National Fibromyalgia & Chronic Pain Association. Hydrocodone rescheduling survey preliminary results. 2015. Available at: http://www.fmcpaware.org/hydrocodone-rescheduling-survey-preliminary-results.html. Accessed October 15, 2015.
55. Nuckols TK, Anderson L, Popescu I, et al. Opioid prescribing: a systematic review and critical appraisal of guidelines for chronic pain. Ann Intern Med 2014;160:38–47.
56. Chou R, Fanciullo GJ, Fine PG, et al. Clinical guidelines for the use of chronic opioid therapy in chronic noncancer pain. J Pain 2009;10:113–30. Available at: http://www.ncbi.nlm.nih.gov/pubmed/19187889. Accessed October 13, 2015.
57. Kahan M, Mailis-Gagnon A, Wilson L, et al, National Opioid Use Guideline Group. Canadian guideline for safe and effective use of opioids for chronic noncancer pain: clinical summary for family physicians. Part 1: general population. Can Fam Physician 2011;57:1257–66, e407–18. Available at: http://www.ncbi.nlm.nih.gov/pubmed/22084455. Accessed October 27, 2015.
58. Kahan M, Wilson L, Mailis-Gagnon A, et al, National Opioid Use Guideline Group. Canadian guideline for safe and effective use of opioids for chronic noncancer pain: clinical summary for family physicians. Part 2: special populations. Can Fam Physician 2011;57:1269–76, e419–28. Available at: http://www.ncbi.nlm.nih.gov/pubmed/22084456. Accessed October 27, 2015.
59. Webster LR, Webster RM. Predicting aberrant behaviors in opioid-treated patients: preliminary validation of the opioid risk tool. Pain Med 2005;6:432–42.

60. Butler SF, Budman SH, Fernandez K, et al. Validation of a screener and opioid assessment measure for patients with chronic pain. Pain 2004;112:65–75.

61. Butler SF, Fernandez K, Benoit C, et al. Validation of the revised screener and opioid assessment for patients with pain (SOAPP-R). J Pain 2008;9:360–72.

62. Belgrade MJ, Schamber CD, Lindgren BR. The DIRE score: predicting outcomes of opioid prescribing for chronic pain. J Pain 2006;7:671–81.

63. Passik SD, Kirsh KL, Whitcomb L, et al. Monitoring outcomes during long-term opioid therapy for noncancer pain: results with the pain assessment and documentation tool. J Opioid Manag 2005;1:257–66, 423.

64. Butler SF, Budman SH, Fernandez KC, et al. Development and validation of the current opioid misuse measure. Pain 2007;130:144–56.

65. Federation of State Medical Boards of the United States, Inc. Model policy on the use of opioid analgesics in the treatment of chronic pain. Washington, DC: Federation of State Medical Boards; 2013. Available at: http://www.fsmb.org/Media/Default/PDF/FSMB/Advocacy/pain_policy_july2013.pdf. Accessed October 19, 2015.

66. Peles E, Schreiber S, Gordon J, et al. Significantly higher methadone dose for methadone maintenance treatment (MMT) patients with chronic pain. Pain 2005;113:340–6.

67. Potter JS, Shiffman SJ, Weiss RD. Chronic pain severity in opioid-dependent patients. Am J Drug Alcohol Abuse 2008;34:101–7.

68. Rosenblum A, Joseph H, Fong C, et al. Prevalence and characteristics of chronic pain among chemically dependent patients in methadone maintenance and residential treatment facilities. JAMA 2003;289:2370–8.

69. Sheu R, Lussier D, Rosenblum A, et al. Prevalencnt drug and alcohol treatment program. Pain Med 2008;9:911–7.

70. National Institute on Drug Abuse. Comorbidity: addiction and other mental illness. Research report series. NIH publication No. 10-5771. 2010. Available at: https://www.drugabuse.gov/publications/research-reports/comorbidity-addiction-other-mental-illnesses/letter-director. Accessed October 27, 2015.

71. Goldberg DS. On the erroneous conflation of opiophobia and the undertreatment of pain. Am J Bioeth 2010;10:20–2.

Advancing the Pain Agenda in the Veteran Population

Rollin M. Gallagher, MD, MPH[a,b]

KEYWORDS

- Pain • Chronification • Stepped care • Opioids • Veterans • Biopsychosocial
- JPEP • Mini-residency

KEY POINTS

- Pain is more prevalent and more complex in Veterans whose wounds from severe injuries, including blasts, are also frequently complicated by posttraumatic stress disorder and traumatic brain injury.
- Pain management should begin as soon as possible after injury to prevent the chronification of pain.
- Pain management should be continuous and multimodal, reflecting the influence of somatic, psychological, and social factors on pain perception, psychological response, and treatment outcomes.
- The Stepped Care Model is an evidence-based approach to providing patient-centered biopsychosocial pain care at the level of the veteran's needs based on complexity, comorbidity, refractoriness, and risk.
- Methods to provide outcomes measurement to assist real-time clinical decision making are needed.

INTRODUCTION: PAIN, A PUBLIC HEALTH PROBLEM

Pain leadership in the Veterans Health Administration (VHA) has outlined 6 essential elements of effective pain management (**Box 1**). Its efforts to be successful in implementing these elements system-wide are outlined in this article. Transforming pain care in the VHA occurs in the context of a gradual, decades-old cultural shift in attitudes toward pain in the United States and globally. Although chronic pain has been identified as a public health problem by our field for at least 2 decades,[1–3] only recently has chronic pain been presented in more public-facing media as a national and global health burden. The *Economist's* recent article on global disability[4]

This paper does not reflect the official views of the Department of Veterans Affairs.
[a] Pain Service, Michael Crescenz VA Medical Center, University and Woodland, Philadelphia, PA 19035, USA; [b] Penn Pain Medicine, University of Pennsylvania, Philadelphia, PA, USA
E-mail addresses: rollin.gallagher@va.gov; rgallagh@mail.med.upenn.edu

Anesthesiology Clin 34 (2016) 357–378
http://dx.doi.org/10.1016/j.anclin.2016.01.003   **anesthesiology.theclinics.com**
1932-2275/16/$ – see front matter Published by Elsevier Inc.

Box 1
The 6 steps to good chronic pain care

Outlining the challenge: transforming VA pain care

1. Educate Veterans/families and promote self-efficacy

2. Educate/train all team members

3. Develop nonpharmacologic modalities

4. Institute safe medication prescribing, including safe opioid use (universal precautions)

5. Develop approaches to bringing the veteran's expanded team together (virtual pain consulting and education as well as ongoing communication between team members)

6. Establish metrics to monitor pain care

From U.S. Department of Veterans Affairs. VHA Pain Management. 2015. Available at: http://www.va.gov/painmanagement/. Accessed December 21, 2015.

---

discussed the economic implications of a study by the World Health Organization[5] implicating low back pain as the most common cause of disability worldwide, including in North America, South America, Europe, Australia, Indonesia, and most of Asia. Low back pain and other chronic pain syndromes, such as the most common disabling disease in South Africa, human immunodeficiency virus/AIDS, are commonly comorbid with and precede depression, which is the most common disabling condition in several of the most populous African and South American countries and in India and Pakistan.

In the United States, the concept of pain as a major public health problem gained traction in a wider sector of American society during the last decade, fueled by 3 intersecting societal problems discussed in Congress and academic and health policy circles and covered in the press.

First, hundreds of thousands of American troops were returning home with painful conditions from the Middle East for care in military and the Department of Veterans Affairs (VA) facilities, many with comorbidities, such as posttraumatic stress disorder (PTSD) and postconcussive syndrome; as substance abuse and suicide rates increased in this population, pain was discovered to be a driving factor.[6–8]

Second, economic studies suggested how chronic pain contributed to our nation's increasing health care costs and impacted the competiveness of America's businesses and overall economic health[9] (Institute of Medicine [IOM] 2010).

Third, the increasing rates of prescription analgesic drug abuse and overdose deaths and its impact on public health[10–12] in the general population and in Veterans and service members raised national awareness of the importance of effective and safe pain management.

Although organized medicine, beset with its increasing costs and inefficient systems, had been unable to address the public health problem of pain, patients and their families spoke up and Congress listened, passing 3 pain bills: (1) the Veterans Pain Care Act (2008)[13]; (2) the Military Pain Care Act (2009),[14] both requiring yearly progress reports from these agencies; and (3) on the coattails of these first two bills, the requirement in the 2010 Patient Protection and Affordable Care Act (2010)[15] that the IOM complete a national study of pain. The IOM study documented that about 100 million adults (approximately 30% of American adults) have some form of chronic pain and that the cost of chronic pain, $565 to $635 billion yearly, exceeds the combined costs of cancer and heart disease.[9] The IOM's report cited myriad actions required to begin addressing this enormous public health problem, including the following:

- Health care provider organizations should promote and enable self-management of pain as the starting point of management.
  - Develop educational approaches and culturally and linguistically appropriate materials to promote and enable self-management.
- Population strategy should include developing strategies to overcome barriers to care.
  - Strategies should focus on ways to improve care for populations disproportionately affected by and undertreated for pain.
- Health professions' education and training programs, professional associations, and other groups should provide educational opportunities in pain assessment and treatment in primary care.
  - Education should improve knowledge and skills in pain assessment and treatment.
- Pain specialty professional organizations and primary care professional associations should support collaboration between pain specialists and primary care clinicians, including greater proficiency by primary care providers (PCPs) along with referral to pain centers when appropriate.
- Payers and health care organizations should revise reimbursement policies to foster coordinated and evidence-based pain care.
- Health care providers should provide consistent and complete pain assessments.

PAIN IN MILITARY PERSONNEL AND IN VETERANS

Although about 30% of the US adult population experiences chronic pain, the rate in Veterans enrolled in the VHA is much higher. In older Veterans, the rate approaches 50%[16]; their pain tends to be more complex, with higher rates of psychiatric and social comorbidities, such as substance abuse, depression, PTSD, and early work disability. This rate has grown steadily over the last 2 decades as aging warriors from earlier military service have retired and sought VA care for chronic illness management that the VA excels at providing relative to the general health sector. They bring with them pain from service-related and battlefield injuries as well as pain from the diseases and their treatments associated with aging, such as cancer, arthritis, spinal conditions, and neuropathies. The survivors of war, such as those who served in Vietnam, also suffer its mental health consequences, with higher rates than the general population for PTSD and other mental scars of exposure to the battlefield.

Rates of pain are even higher in VA enrollees from the recent Middle Eastern wars. Almost 60% have musculoskeletal conditions, such as lower back pain.[17] More serious injuries, such as penetrating wounds and mine blasts, that had low survival in Vietnam (40%), now lead to 90% survival because of advances in personal battlefield armor and combat casualty care. These Veterans enter the VHA with permanently damaged, painful musculoskeletal tissues and peripheral nerves, including amputations and spinal cord injuries, and often with several somatic and neuropathic sources of pain[18–22] that affect longitudinal function.[23] All Veterans with battlefield exposure risk PTSD from their exposure to the dangers and horrors of war. Those exposed to blasts may have traumatic brain injury with high rates of pain and PTSD together (54%) and pain alone (70%).[24,25] Collectively these conditions impact Veterans' longer-term physical, emotional and social well-being, as well as their successful reintegration to family and community life and lead to consequences, such as depression, substance use disorder (SUD), disability, overdose, and suicide.

An additional problem related to pain management facing the nation and the Department of Defense (DoD) and VA, the greatly increased availability of opioids, has contributed to the opioid epidemic of increasing overdose rates.[26] This epidemic has many causes.[10] The VHA, which unlike the private sector has the capacity to study its deidentified administrative database for a complete sample of all enrolled Veterans, has conducted some of the studies identifying factors that increase risks for overdose, such as higher daily doses, coprescription of benzodiazepines, and the comorbidities of SUD, depression, and PTSD.[10–12,27] This database also provides the opportunity for studying the impact of an intervention, such as the Opioid Safety Initiative (which is discussed later), to address such a public health problem.

THE PREVENTION AND REVERSAL OF PAIN CHRONIFICATION

Animal studies detailing the neurobiology of the development of chronic pain following injury, and human studies detailing the clinical course of pain after injury, have led to a new modeling of pain's progression from acute to chronic pain, termed *chronification*.[27–30] **Fig. 1**, the chronification cycle,[31] simplistically diagrams the complicated phenomenological process involved in the longitudinal course of pain and its consequences. **Fig. 1** suggests that an effective health care system must have the capacity for timely intervention at each stage to minimize the chances of progression to pathologic structural and neurobehavioral changes and attendant social morbidities, as well as to treat and, whenever possible, to reverse them.

Primary Prevention

The focus in primary prevention is that of actively shifting attitudes toward health, through engagement in healthy activities and lifestyles that prevent pain-causing

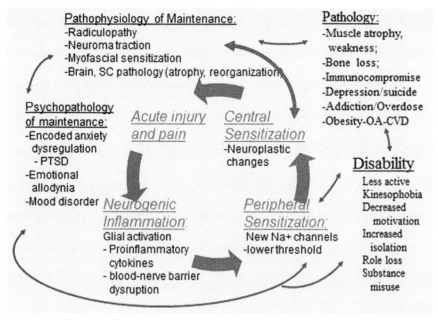

Fig. 1. Chronification of pain and the chronic pain cycle. OA-CVD, osteoarthritis, cardiovascular disease; SC, spinal cord. (*From* Gallagher RM. Management strategies for chronic pain. In: Krames ES, Peckham PH, Rezai AR, editors. Neuromodulation. New York: Academic Press; 2009. p. 315; with permission.)

disease and injury. The use of protective devices against injuries such as body armor and seat-belts, smoking avoidance and cessation, weight control, exercise, and forms of stress management (eg, yoga, meditation) are conceptualized. Establishing a platform of sound health practices provides a self-management foundation for longitudinally effective pain care.

Secondary Prevention

The focus in secondary prevention is on effective pain care after injury/disease onset. Care aims to

- Avoid unnecessary pain and secondary sensitization of the central nervous system (CNS) through peripheral pain control with timely application of neuromodulation (eg, ice, transcutaneous electrical nerve stimulation, neurostimulators), medications, and neural blockade with regional anesthesia.
- Reduce central pain perception and suffering through appropriate and safe use of medication and self-management techniques.
- Reduce structural and neurobehavioral damage from the injury itself and from its treatment (eg, surgery, chemotherapy/radiotherapy, medication toxicities).
- Promote healing and disease modification to restore and maintain a person's function and quality of life, including support from family and community.

Tertiary Prevention

The focus of tertiary prevention is functional restoration when a painful condition persists and becomes a chronic nociceptive or neuropathic stimulus leading to pain chronification. Treatments target pathophysiologic neuroplastic changes to the spinal cord and brain affecting pain perception, emotions, cognition, and maladaptive behaviors. Early recognition, prevention, and management of mood, sleep, and SUDs are key objectives.

As suggested in **Fig. 1**, the course of chronification is determined by a person's somatic pain condition interacting with their emotions and interpersonal and physical environments, including their health care system. The behavioral neuroscience of this interaction underpins the principles of designing and assembling a health system that provides safe and effective pain care to a population.

- Once the pain-causing disease process or injury is effectively managed, and pain treatment commences, the salience of emotions and the social environment to pain perception and behavior becomes apparent.
- Pain is powerfully conditioning, and its relief is highly rewarding; whoever and whatever achieves that relief is greatly appreciated by the organism. Simply put as follows:
  - Actions that bring relief are highly reinforced. Thus, when a movement hurts, the brain automatically says *do not move again* or *move in a way that does not hurt*; and the pain does not occur or is relieved if it did occur. The pain ceases or is avoided when the organism does not move that way. This sequence activates the reward centers in the brain and is remembered. Thus, patients need instruction in healthy movement and reinforcement for learning to overcome the fear of healthy movement, even if it activates pain no longer directly related to the ongoing tissue injury or disease.
  - Similarly when a medication, such as an opioid, reliably relieves the pain, the effect of that rewarding experience is the motivation to use it again when the stimulus recurs or the brain's opioid level decrease, unmasking the painful stimulus.

- Patients with SUD, or a genetic predisposition, are vulnerable to the rewarding characteristics of the opioid molecule on top of the reward of pain relief. This characteristic may lead to continued and increased use, even when the pain stimulus is well controlled or is eliminated. Hence, an effective care system must both identify such predisposition and provide closer monitoring.
  - Other pathways may also promote the chronification process, such as neurogenesis-dependent, hippocampal-associative learning mechanisms that are known to be associated with emergence of persistent pain from acute pain, and the interaction of depression with pain.[32]
- The clinical care system must be designed to account for the reality that not all chronic pain is the same. People differ in the peripheral stimulus, their CNS-mediated response to the activation of pain, the reward of pain relief, and the reward of opioids (particularly for those with SUD). There is also considerable variability in how those within patients' health care system understand and manage those differences in each patient and their respective social network.[33] All of these factors taken together will determine outcomes of treatment. Especially identifying SUD or risk for SUD, and tailoring treatment accordingly, is paramount for good population outcomes.

Knowledge of the framework outlined earlier is essential for developing competency in pain assessment and biopsychosocial formulation and goal-oriented management planning, with an individualized array of choices for each patient and clinician to achieve safe and effective relief and to restore function and quality of life.[34]

The large proportion and sheer number of Veterans with complex pain conditions requires that the VHA and DoD make important structural and process changes in the approach to pain care that assures effective and safe pain management. For example, data suggest that optimal acute pain care after battlefield or other injury might include one or more of the following, each targeting a separate process in the acute pain experience:

- Regional anesthesia for neural blockade shortly after injury to prevent access of the pain stimulus to the CNS[35]
- Early use of ketamine to prevent wind-up and sensitization[36]
- Opioids when needed to reduce suffering and its activation of central stress pathways contributing to chronification[37]
- Cognitive-behavioral/psychophysiologic stress control techniques[38]
- The development of goal-oriented management plans that include[39]
  - Careful longitudinal monitoring to assure safe and appropriate use of medications and other interventions
  - The early integration of behavioral and integrative strategies such as cognitive-behavioral/psychophysiologic training, acupuncture, yoga and meditation
  - Careful transition plans from hospital care to outpatient care
  - Effective communication about the plan of care and key information in the transition of care to the VA and/or community clinicians following discharge from the DoD

STRUCTURAL CHALLENGES

The VA's obligations to its Veterans required immediate and sustainable transformative changes in pain management in a population-based, public health approach to the management of pain; support for the health system's research is needed to guide implementation. There are no easy solutions and many challenges in designing and implementing an effective, population-based model of pain care in a health system.

The VHA and the private health system are burdened by

- Inadequately trained workforces in pain management, including both primary care and specialists[9,40]
- The lack of clinical practice guidelines/algorithms that are supported by good evidence, particularly combined treatments that can be used in primary care
- Poor fiscal support or credit for effective nonmedical pain management interventions
- Measuring quality by volume and number of procedures rather than clinical outcomes
- Interspecialty competition for lucrative procedures associated with specialty care, impeding cooperation and collaboration

VHA's challenges that differ from the private health care system include the following:

- It has a capitated system with fixed budgets that precludes the following:
  - Development of profit centers that in the private system generate revenue, with personnel recruitment affected by lower salaries
  - A business model allowing for a quick response to rapid *increases* in demand such as occurred following 9/11 and the subsequent wars that created hundreds of thousands of new Veterans with pain and comorbidities
- It has an obligation to care for all Veterans (ie, no cherry picking of cases); clinical teams must care for all cases, regardless of complexity. They cannot be discharged from care as they might be in private practice where insurance for behavioral treatments of vexing comorbidities is limited. Thus, more complex patients tend to selectively seek the VHA for their care and are a higher time and cost burden.
- Public scrutiny supports health systems research that finds flaws in care and gaps in the VA's health delivery and publishes those findings in the lay press and in medical journals.[41] Although this level of transparency eventually may spur system interventions to correct problems, these reports bring negative congressional and constituent attention to the VA.

The VHA's advantages over private health systems include the following:

- Administrative databases and the electronic medical record provide complete samples of its patient population to discover gaps in care and also provide baseline data for outcome studies of system interventions to correct gaps.[42–44]
- Decisions about system design and clinical processes are not pressured to generate income to the degree they are in the private health sector, providing greater opportunity for studying innovations and, if successful, their system-wide deployment.
- The National Pain Management Strategy Coordinating Committee (NPMSCC) (**Box 2**), with representatives from all relevant VHA national offices, supports a National Pain Management Program (NPMP) office that advises the VHA on pain management policy and implementation.
- It has a workforce self-selected to be mission focused, not income focused. In the VHA many clinicians prefer the teamwork and support for good pain care that is sometimes harder to achieve in a private or university setting where generating revenue is paramount.

Box 2
The NPMSCC (Field Advisory Committee)

National Pain Program office: director, deputy director, research advisor, program coordinator

- Primary care[2]
- Physical Medicine and Rehabilitation
- Pain medicine[2]
- Addictions
- Neurology
- Mental health integration
- Pain psychology
- Patient education
- Anesthesiology
- Geriatrics
- Postdeployment health[2]
- Pharmacy (Pharmacy Benefits Management)
- Nursing[2]
- Employee Education System[2]
- Women's health
- Research
- Integrated health

- There is no reinforcement of the models of pain care in the community that perpetuate fragmented, ineffective care[45,46]:
  - *The sequential specialty/subspecialty care model*: Patients with pain are referred among specialists seeking to find and eliminate the somatic pain source with more tests and procedures without formulating the dynamic interaction of biopsychosocial factors, translated through behavioral neuroscience, that influence the course and outcomes of any one patient's pain. Chronification occurs and costs accrue.
  - *The multidisciplinary pain center model*: Patients fail traditional, sequential care, at high cost, including disability, facilitating chronification and its consequences and are then referred to a costly program to reverse chronification and its morbidities.[47]
  - *The managed care model*: Access to pain medicine specialty team care is not available or if available is limited to costly procedures, not expert biopsychosocial care. They tend to be placed on escalating doses of medications, such as opioids, with their complications and, because of ineffective care, are often unable to return to work or other role functioning.
- VHA has the ability to adopt new models of care delivery that promise to address these structural, socioeconomic, and clinical process issues in a community or health system caring for a defined population of patients. To this end, a new model of care is proposed: the Pain Medicine and Primary Care Community Rehabilitation Model (PMPCCRM).[45,46] This model is designed to emphasize the critical role of clinical teams in a community, anchored by competent PCPs with access to pain medicine specialty teams in that community.

○ *PCPs* and their clinical teams add expert evidence-based pain management clinical algorithms for pain management to their skills in longitudinal, comprehensive chronic care.[48–52] Combined with their more intimate knowledge of general health maintenance and management techniques, family and other psychosocial factors, and community resources that might importantly influence the outcome of pain treatment, PCPs can tailor a biopsychosocial care plan that is individualized to their patients' respective needs.[34]

○ *Pain medicine specialty teams,* including integrative, behavioral, and physical therapies, actively collaborate with a community's primary care network to be easily accessible for consultation and specialty treatment to reduce chronification when PCP treatment is ineffective.

○ *Interdisciplinary pain rehabilitation centers,* in the CARF model, are accessible when, despite the collaboration of primary care and pain medicine teams, chronification progresses to disability and its related comorbidities.

THE STEPPED-CARE APPROACH

In response to these challenges and building on the principles of the PMPCCRM, the VHA has designed a population-based, stepped approach to pain management that focuses on primary, secondary, and tertiary prevention. A progression of activities led to the publication and dissemination in 2009 of a policy directive, written by this author and Dr Robert Kerns, then the National Pain Director, with the support and input of pain colleagues and the interprofessional NPMSCC representing various clinical offices in the VHA (see **Box 1**). The directive[53] outlined a new standard of care for pain for the entire VA, Stepped Pain Care, which directed that a biopsychosocial model of patient-centered chronic pain care be provided seamlessly and collaboratively in primary care, secondary care, and tertiary care with movement between sectors depending on complexity, treatment refractoriness, comorbidities, and risk as illustrated in **Fig. 2**. This model is consistent with the medical home model in the Affordable Care Act in that it requires the partnership of informed patients and a proactive health care system that is designed to engage patients in their health care planning and decisions. The model emphasizes the value of interdisciplinary teamwork in providing biopsychosocial, patient-centered pain management in primary care with easy access to consultation and collaborative models of care with necessary specialists, particularly an interdisciplinary pain specialty team, and underpinned by a strong institutional culture of a shared mission and responsibility.

To fully implement a public health model of pain management in its target populations, the VA must work closely with the DoD, within whose sphere (combat) pain usually starts. In 2009 Lieutenant General Dr Eric Schoomaker, the Army Surgeon General, chartered the Army Pain Task Force, including pain experts from the Army, Navy, and Air Force, with the author representing the VA. The Task Force completed an intensive, 6-month, in-depth study of pain management in the military, making dozens of site visits to highly reputed practices as well as holding 3 retreats, and published a 163-page report,[54] which thoroughly outlined the current deficiencies in care. From these activities and insights, the group made more than 100 recommendations for transforming pain care in the military. Key among these was the adoption of the VHA's Stepped Care Model of pain management. Subsequently, the VA-DoD Health Executive Council (HEC), cochaired by their undersecretaries for health, chartered a Pain Management Working Group (HEC-PMWG), cochaired by this author and Dr Chester (Trip) Buckenmaier, which was charged with establishing a single system of continuous, collaborative, and effective pain care, research, and education for the

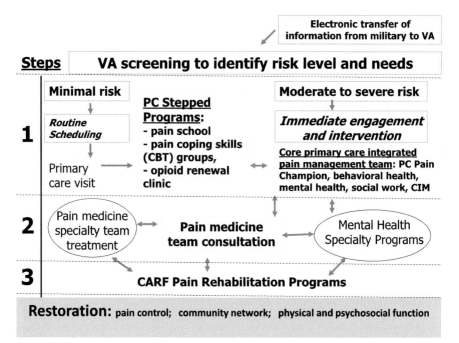

Fig. 2. Continuum of VHA stepped pain care. CBT, cognitive behavioral therapy; CIM, complementary and integrative medicine; PC, primary care. (*From* Gallagher RM. Pain medicine and primary care: the evolution of a population-based approach to chronic pain as a public health problem. In: Deer TR, Leong MS, Buvanendran A, et al, editors. Comprehensive treatment of chronic pain by medical, interventional, and behavioral approaches. The American Academy of Pain Medicine textbook on patient management. New York: Springer; 2013; with permission. "Comprehensive Treatment of Chronic Pain by Medical, Interventional, and Behavioral Approaches. The American Academy of Pain Medicine Textbook on Patient Management" is a copyrighted work of the American Academy of Pain Medicine. © American Academy of Pain Medicine 2013.)

VA and DoD. The Defense and Veterans Center for Integrated Pain Management is a newly functional office chartered under the lead of the Army, and now under the Uniform Services University of the Health Sciences, to help operationalize the work of the HEC-PMWG.[55]

Early descriptions of the VA's Stepped Care Model[56] have been updated with an increased emphasis on teaching self-management[57] as well as system support for primary care by pharmacists through medication and opioid management.[58,59] Also added are behavioral health technicians for screening and management of aberrant illness behavior and mental health comorbidities[60,61] and access to evidence-based guidelines and clinical algorithms.[48–52,62] The evidence base for this model is emerging from clinical trials and cohort studies in primary care systems. Notably, all of these have been conducted in the VHA, wherein specific primary care enhancements have been shown to improve outcomes in primary care practices managing pain. Examples of these stepped programs include the following:

- Dobcha and colleagues,[42] in a blinded cluster-randomized controlled trial, compared the impact of an 'assistance with pain treatments' intervention with 'treatment as usual' in 401 Veterans with musculoskeletal pain cared for by 42 primary care physicians over a 12-month period. They found significant improvements in pain disability, patients' ratings of global impression of change, and depression severity in those with depression.

- Kroenke and colleagues[63] completed a randomized controlled study (Stepped Care for Affective Disorders and Musculoskeletal Pain) of the impact of a 12-week stepped program versus treatment as usual in Veterans with musculoskeletal pain and depression. The stepped program, consisting of optimized antidepressant therapy and participation in a pain self-management program, substantially improved depression and moderately reduce pain severity and disability.
- Wiedemer and colleagues[58,59] studied the impact of creating a structured pharmacist-run clinic for Veterans with aberrant behavior, when prescribed opioids in a primary care setting. Almost half of those referred with aberrant behavior and all those with risk factors for abuse without aberrancy could be managed effectively. The use of urine drug screens for patients on long-term opioids in primary care increased significantly, and provider satisfaction was high.
- Bair and colleagues's[64] study Evaluation of Stepped Care for Chronic Pain in Veterans of the Iraq-Afghanistan war with musculoskeletal pain found that the combination of algorithm-guided analgesics, self-management training, and brief cognitive behavioral therapy provided by trained nurses resulted in significant improvements in pain severity as well as in pain-related disability and interference.

To promote this transformation in all 142 VHA medical facilities and their related outpatient clinics, the VHA established an NPMP office, which is responsible for policy development, coordination, oversight, and monitoring of the VHA National Pain Management Strategy in collaboration with other relevant VHA program offices, such as primary care, mental health, pharmacy benefits management services, nursing, integrative health, and the other national offices and programs listed in **Box 1**.

The NPMP is supported by and supports several task forces in addition to the NPMSCC now cochaired by Drs. Friedhelm Sandbrink and Robert Sproul, and work groups that enable VHA to achieve its goal of implementing a patient-aligned, Stepped Care Model of team-based pain care system-wide. Monthly meetings include the following:

- NPMSCC (see **Box 1**) for advice and support from the other VA clinical and operational offices monthly
- The National Pain Leadership Group consisting of 22 Veterans Integrated Service Network (VISN) (regional) and 142 facility Pain Points of Contact with whom new VA Central Office (VACO) programs and policies are shared and who provide feedback to VACO from the field
- The Primary Care Task Force that supports the Primary Care Pain Team (PACT) Pain Champions in the facilities across the system
- The interdisciplinary Pain Medicine Specialty Team Work Group that aims to standardize accessible, effective, pain specialty consultation and collaboration and referrals to Step 2 across the system[65]
- The CARF Pain Rehabilitation Task Force that provides training and standardization of CARF functions across the system[66,67]

National, regional, and facility responsibilities within the VHA network are outlined in the VHA Pain Management Directive 2009-053,[53] which, besides outlining the Stepped Care Model, requires the following:

- Standards for education and training that would generate a clinical workforce with the competencies needed to provide good pain care

- A system of monitoring care system-wide to assure safety and effectiveness
- A system of identifying quality improvement and implementation research successes to develop evidence-based stepped care strong practices or bright spots
- A system of communicating about such practices and for implementing them system-wide

PROVIDING EDUCATION AND TRAINING

To inform the field of challenges, goals, and plans, late in the last decade VHA conducted national and regional workshops for pain champions and pain experts from regions (VISNs) and facilities across the country. Following recommendations[9,40] that training improve both in postgraduate and graduate medical education, a VHA workgroup identified core competencies for VHA PCPs in pain management, as listed in **Table 1**, now further developed by national workgroups.[48–52,60,68–70] Programs to address these competencies encompass office-based procedures and interventions, such as taught by the VHA's Pain Mini-Residency.[71]

The VHA and DoD have developed several national education and training programs to improve the pain management competencies of its present and future work force.

- VA-DoD Tiered Acupuncture Training Across Clinical Settings aims to train physicians in medical acupuncture and providers in battlefield (auricular) acupuncture (BFA) across both DoD and VA health systems, so that Veterans have access to acupuncture as a first-line treatment of pain.[72,73] Already, training has occurred for several thousand front-line clinicians in battlefield acupuncture and for almost 100 medical acupuncturists in a 300-hour course, leading to them becoming BFA faculty (instructors) who are distributed across the health system to sustain the expansion of this workforce so all Veterans will eventually have access.
- VA-DoD Joint Pain Education Project (JPEP): JPEP[74] convened subject matter experts in the broad domains of pain management knowledge and skills to create a virtual textbook of 27 modules of evidence-based instruction in pain management. These modules are released for use in all VA-DoD educational programs, such as Specialty Care Access Network (SCAN) Extension for Community Healthcare Outcomes (ECHO), the Mini-Residency, and asynchronous online trainings; integration into medical residency programs and other professional training programs has begun. (The VA provides full or partial training to about 70% of US-trained physicians.)
- Pain Mini-Residency for PCPs: This curriculum[71] emphasizes the development of competencies in history, physical examination, and goal-oriented biopsychosocial treatment planning for common regional pain syndromes. Important components of the development of PCPs' skills include the following:
  - Recognizing when and how to treat a given condition using an array of medical, behavioral, and integrated health treatment options, including training in specific office-based procedures, such as BFA and trigger point injections
  - Recognizing when and how to make appropriate referrals to a specialty care pain service
  - Learning the communication skills to effectively discuss a biopsychosocial plan of care with Veterans
  - The program uses instructional materials from an approved standardized national curriculum (JPEP) and includes a virtual learning phase, a 3-day face-to-face component, and a follow-up preceptor phase using existing training

Table 1
Core competencies in primary care pain management

Primary Care Competency	Educational Strategy	Measurement of Achievement	Strategies for Sustainability

• Conduct of comprehensive pain assessment
  ○ History including assessment of psychiatric/behavioral comorbidities, addiction, and aberrant behavior (diversion)
  ○ Conduct of routine focused physical/neurologic examinations
  ○ Judicious use of diagnostic tests/procedures
	• Web-based training
	• In-person training sessions
	• Manuals from Pain.Edu
		• Completion of training (mini-residency, SCAN ECHO, TMS) (asynchronous)
		• Chart review
			• Panel size adjustments and increased visit time for pain patients
			• Performance measures/monitors
			• PACT pain champions

• Optimal patient communication
  ○ How to encourage realistic evidence-based expectations
  ○ How to provide reassurance and discourage negative behavior
  ○ How to foster pain self-management
  ○ Negotiating behaviorally specific and feasible goals
	• Web-based training
	• In-person training sessions
	• Manuals from Pain.Edu
	• Motivational interview training
		• Completion of training
		• Patient feedback
		• Patient satisfaction surveys, but must account for skew due to disgruntled patients, secondary gain
		• Ongoing reassessment of treatment plan
		• Appropriately soliciting patient questions and concerns
			• Availability of wellness programs
			• Behavioral management/pain psychology
			• Patient support groups
			• Templates for functional evaluation and reevaluation
			• PACT pain champions

• Pain management
  ○ Knowledge of accepted clinical practice guidelines
  ○ Rational, algorithmic-based polypharmacy and goal-oriented biopsychosocial care plans
  ○ Institute safe and effective opioid management procedures
  ○ Knowledge/use of common metrics for measuring function
  ○ Determining the need for stepped care with behavioral, integrative health, and physical therapies and integrating them into care plans appropriately
  ○ Determining the need for secondary consultation and creating functional consultation and collaborative care processes
	• Web-based training
	• In-person training sessions
	• Manuals pain Web site
	• List of available services
	• Service agreements
	• Web-based info on local arrangements
	• Links to practice guidelines
	• Use of Academic Detailing Program
		• Completion of training
		• Medication utilization monitoring (long-acting vs short-acting opioids, nonopioid therapy)
		• Utilization of adjuvant therapy, other interventions
		• Chart review
			• Separate problem patients from regular PC pain population
			• Identify and review outliers
			• Availability of wellness/integrative health programs
			• Behavioral management/pain psychology
			• Performance measures/monitors
			• PACT pain champions

Abbreviations: PACT, patient aligned care team; TMS, talent management system.

programs, such as SCAN ECHO, academic detailing, and local preceptor instruction and support.

- Pain SCAN-ECHO: The VHA's pain management SCAN ECHO[44] program derives from the University of New Mexico's ECHO model of using videoconferencing technology to teach providers chronic pain management skills beyond that of their previous training.[75] In the model of a resident case conference, interdisciplinary teams of clinicians (pain medicine specialists, pain psychologists, psychiatrists, social workers, pharmacists, integrative health clinicians, and physical therapists) simultaneously supervise several providers whose patients have difficulty accessing specialty pain care because of one or more factors, such as distance, transportation, and illness severity. Using checklists for gathering standard clinical information regarding the patients' condition, the pain specialty team helps providers complete an assessment and develop an individualized treatment plan that, in turn, is then tracked at important milestones unless an urgent/emergent issue arises. The specialty team and PCP will modify the treatment plan as needed. A didactic presentation (professional education credit included) related to the cases presented accompanies each session. Ultimately, the program aims to create a knowledge network, with ECHO trainees in the primary care site having a force multiplier effect that improves the pain management skills of other clinicians in their setting. SCAN ECHO, which is particularly beneficial in rural and underserved geographic areas where Veterans have low access to pain specialty care, has been adopted in 6 different regions of the VHA. Benefits of this program include the following:
  - Reduced travel burden by delivering pain management closer to Veterans' homes
  - Lower utilization of specialty care
  - Improved quality of care through PCPs' development of clinical competencies in pain management
    - Early results, comparing 2 similar hub and spoke systems in the VHA, one with SCAN-ECHO and the other without, demonstrated that providers who participated in Pain SCAN-ECHO showed increased use of nonopioid pain medications and physical therapy.[44]
  - Higher provider and veteran satisfaction
- Opioid Safety Initiative (OSI): The OSI[76] project monitors targeted safety practices in opioid pain management, such as reductions in prescribing high-dose opioids and opioids and benzodiazepines together, and increases in use of urine drug screens and evidence-based nonmedical therapies, such as cognitive behavioral therapy and complementary and integrative health treatments, both which are now required to be available in all facilities. Several projects support OSI.
  - OSI toolkit: An expert, interdisciplinary team provides detailed, evidence-based, and peer-reviewed education and guidance for both providers and patients. The toolkit, with public-facing materials available on the VA's Pain Management Internet site[77] and clinician-facing materials on the VA's Pain Management Intranet site, has been widely presented throughout the VHA in multiple educational formats and communications. For example, the toolkit has detailed instructions about guiding safe medication tapers from opioids when clinically indicated. Besides clinical guidance, interested readers can find many other public-facing assets in the toolkit.
  - Signature informed consent for long-term opioid prescribing: VHA Directive 1005, Informed Consent for Long-term Opioid Therapy for Pain, ensures that all Veterans on long-term opioids (more than 3 months and not for palliative or cancer care) have an informed discussion with their prescriber and

health care team on the risks and benefits of chronic opioids for the management of chronic pain and alternative therapies for pain. This discussion is guided by a detailed review of the document, "Taking Opioids Responsibly."[78] This approach standardizes the essentials of safe opioid prescribing in VHA by normalizing provider-veteran discussions and the use of routine urine drug screens and by fostering shared decision making about pain management options and medication safety. Many Veterans find the process most helpful when presented in groups whereby discussion is encouraged in a supportive environment that tends to destigmatize the process.

- Opioid Therapy Risk Report: To further strengthen the OSI by supporting clinicians in clinical decision making, the VA recently accelerated the deployment of a state-of-the-art dashboard tool, the Opioid Therapy Risk Report (OTRR) for Veterans prescribed long-term opioids.[79] Dashboards appearing directly in the VHA electronic medical record provide clinicians with point-of-care (real-time) access to veteran-specific data and information. OTRR provides clinician/team point-of-care access to a dashboard for data on each individual veteran's pain-related diagnoses, clinic visits, opioids prescribed, last urine drug screens, psychiatric comorbidities, and completion of the informed consent document. Thus, the OTRR supports providers' panel management and care coordination as well as supporting safe opioid prescribing.

- Academic detailing: One of the major benefits of clinical pain practice in the VHA is the important and growing role of pharmacists trained in pain management as active members of the clinical pain team in facilities. One such project, the Opioid Renewal Clinic,[58] has been described and replicated as Pharmacy Pain Management Clinics across the VHA. Another project is the Academic Detailing (AD) Service,[80] established by the Pharmacy Benefits Management Office to support the Opioid and Psychotropic Drug Safety Initiatives. AD creates and provides patient- and provider-level tools that are designed to be used during AD visits to facilities where AD meets with pain teams and with individual providers needing support to facilitate discussion and address questions related to medications and other treatment modalities. AD is a proven innovation of the academic and private sector to aid in post-training continuing education.[81,82]

- Stratification Tool for Opioid Risk Management (STORM): This project uses the VHA's administrative database to generate data on the effectiveness of the OSI in achieving goals for safer opioid prescribing and by providing evidence as to the impact of specific changes, such as increasing the use of urine drug screens, on reducing risk of opioid overdose.[83]

- Overdose Education and Naloxone Distribution (OEND): This project has created and distributed trainings throughout the VHA promoting awareness of the risks for overdose and training of families and others in the use of naloxone rescue kits to reverse opioid-related overdose. To date, more than 100 potential overdose deaths have been averted.[84]

- Pain nursing: The Pain Management Nursing Work Group, in conjunction with the University of Wisconsin, continues the Pain Resource Nurse (PRN) program,[85] designed specifically to meet the needs of Veterans at all VA sites. Training of nursing pain champions at Tampa VA Medical Center (VAMC) has resulted in trained representatives at 40 VHA facilities. These pain champions are now beginning to develop PRN programs within their local facilities.

VETERANS HEALTH ADMINISTRATION PAIN RESEARCH

The VA's pain research enterprise[86–88] ranges from studies of the neurobiology of disease to implementation research. The nidus of the VA's pain research effort lies in the Pain Research Working Group (PRWG), led by Dr Robert Kerns of VA Connecticut and Yale University in monthly phone meetings for many years and almost yearly in face-to-face meetings in various venues. These meetings facilitate dialogue among pain investigators and the VHA's Office of Research Development and introduce new investigators to the VA pain research enterprise. They foster dialogue and collaborations among VHA investigators and research centers. Dr Kerns, as National Advisor for Pain Research, meets weekly with the National Pain Program office to coordinate discussions with PRWG members about national clinical priorities. The VHA's pain research enterprise addresses our society's important need for implementation research, a recognized donut hole of the National Institutes of Health's research portfolio. The VA's administrative database, built on the electronic health record, enables studies of trends and gaps in care, the effects of larger-scale practice interventions and policy changes, and epidemiologic studies that inform hypotheses for prospective studies, clinical trials, and implementation research. Our research enterprise remains challenged to develop a system of uniform longitudinal pain assessment that provides both meaningful measurement yielding real-time decision support in the clinic as well as building a robust data registry to support large scale studies, although several efforts are presently underway.[89,90]

SUMMARY

Pain management, historically a footnote in the medical battle to cure disease and fix injury, is now being recognized by society as addressing one of its most pressing, longstanding, and costly public health issues. The American people, through their representatives in Congress, now also demand attention to pain; the VA has responded as outlined in this article. The VHA's pain enterprise is vibrant and growing, fueled by the compassion of a workforce dedicated to the mission of relieving the suffering of the men and women who have served our country. The structural problems perpetuating ineffective pain management that are so carefully delineated in the IOM Report[9] have resulted in the Department of Health and Human Services' National Health Strategy,[91] which proposes specific steps in this enterprise, including training and structural changes. Congress asks that we improve the competency of our clinicians and facilities in providing compassionate, safe, and effective care. Working in collaboration with the DoD, the VHA has taken up the challenge of developing effective training, both at the graduate and postgraduate levels. We must now work with our academic partners to ensure the uniform effectiveness of that training system-wide. Similarly, when we demonstrate successful interventions through clinical trials, we must further develop our capacity to implement these interventions system-wide. To achieve our goals, we must support clinicians and their teams as they attempt to engage Veterans in the mission of achieving a health-oriented approach to pain management focused on their function, sense of well-being, and overall quality of life.

ACKNOWLEDGMENTS

The author would like to thank the following VHA leaders, representing hundreds of others across the country, who have committed themselves to the care of pain in our Veterans and to furthering pain management. Cochairs of the NPMSCC: Friedhelm Sandbrink (Deputy National Director), Robert Sproul; Primary Care: Gordon

Schectman, Lucille Burgo, Steven Eraker, Steven Hunt, Ilene Robeck, Peter Marshall, Matt Bair, Erin Krebs, Steve Mudra, Michael Saenger, Pat Dumas; Pain Medicine Specialty Team Work Group: Friedhelm Sandbrink, Sanjog Pangarkar, Aram Mardian, Jack Rosenberg, Michael Craine, Ali Mchaourab, David Drake; Research: Robert Kerns (National Research Advisor), Audrey Kusiak; Anesthesia: John Sum-Ping; DVCIPM/DoD: Chester (Trip) Buckenmaier, Kevin Galloway, Steven Hanling, Chris Spevak, Eric Schoomaker, Richard Thomas; Pharmacy Benefits Management: Mike Valentino, Virginia Torrise, Francine Goodman, Tom Emmendorfer, Michael Chaffman; Academic Detailing: Melissa Christopher, Sarah Popish, Elizabeth Oliva; Mental Health: Dan Kivlahan, Andy Pomerantz, Karen Drexler, Steve Dobcha, Ilse Wiechers, Jodie Trafton; Nursing: Susan Hagen, Jan Elliot, Nancy Wiedemer; Ethics: Ken Berkowitz, Karen Rasmussen, Virginia Sharpe; EES: Anne Turner, Rosemary McIntyre, Anne Sanford; VHA Pain Program office: Pamela Cremo, Merry Dziewit.

REFERENCES

1. Gallagher RM. Chronic pain: a public health problem? Clin J Pain 1998;14(4): 276–8.
2. Gallagher RM. The pain decade and the public health. Pain Med 2000;1(4): 283–5.
3. Cousins MJ, Lynch ME. The declaration Montreal: access to pain management is a fundamental human right. Pain 2011;152(12):2673–4.
4. Burdensome global disability. The Economist 2015. Available at: http://www.economist.com/news/science-and-technology/21654565-global-disability.
5. Global Burden of Disease Study 2013 Collaborators. Global, regional, and national incidence, prevalence, and years lived with disability for 301 acute and chronic diseases and injuries in 188 countries, 1990–2013: a systematic analysis for the Global Burden of Disease Study 2013. Lancet 2015;386(9995):743–800.
6. Cohen SP, Nguyen C, Papoor SG, et al. Back pain during war, an analysis of factors affecting outcome. Arch Intern Med 2009;169(20):1916–23.
7. Gironda RJ, Clark ME, Massengale JP, et al. Pain among veterans of operations Enduring Freedom and Iraqi Freedom. Pain Med 2006;7(4):339–43.
8. Rozanov V, Carli V. Suicide among war veterans. Int J Environ Res Public Health 2012;9(7):2504–19.
9. IOM report: relieving-pain-in-America. Available at: http://www.iom.edu/Reports/2011/Relieving-Pain-in-America-A-Blueprint-for-Transforming-Prevention-Care-Education-Research.aspx. Accessed November 10, 2015.
10. Zedler B, Xie L, Wang L, et al. Risk factors for serious prescription opioid-related toxicity or overdose among Veterans Health Administration patients. Pain Med 2014;15:1911–29.
11. Birnbaum HG, White AG, Schiller M, et al. Societal costs of prescription opioid abuse, dependence, and misuse in the United States. Pain Med 2011;12(4):657–67.
12. Bohnert AS, Valenstein M, Bair MJ, et al. Association between opioid prescribing patterns and opioid overdose-related deaths. JAMA 2011;305(13):1315–21.
13. Veterans Pain Care Act of 2008. Available at: https://www.govtrack.us/congress/bills/110/hr6122. Accessed November 10, 2015.
14. Military Pain Care Act of 2008. Available at: https://www.govtrack.us/congress/bills/110/hr5465. Accessed November 10, 2015.
15. 2010 Patient Protection and Affordable Care Act. Available at: http://www.hhs.gov/healthcare/about-the-law/read-the-law/index.html. Accessed November 10, 2015.

16. Kerns RD, Otis J, Rosenberg R, et al. Veterans' reports of pain and associations with ratings of health, health-risk behaviors, affective distress and use of the healthcare system. JRRD 2003;40(5):371–80.

17. Veterans Health Administration. Analysis of VA health care utilization among Operation Enduring Freedom (OEF), Operation Iraqi Freedom (OIF), and Operation New Dawn (OND) veterans. Washington, DC: Department of Veterans Affairs; 2013.

18. Ficke JR, Pollak AN. Extremity war injuries: development of clinical treatment principles. J Am Acad Orthop Surg 2007;15(10):590–5.

19. Eastridge BJ, Hardin M, Cantrell J, et al. Died of wounds on the battlefield: causation and implications for improving combat casualty care. J Trauma 2011;71(1 Suppl):S4–8.

20. Martin M, Oh J, Currier H, et al. An analysis of in-hospital deaths at a modern combat support hospital. J Trauma 2009;66(4 Suppl):S51–61.

21. Baer D, Dubick MA, Wenke JC, et al. Combat casualty care research at the US Army Institute of Surgical Research. J R Army Med Corps 2009;155(4):327–32.

22. Bridges E, Biever K. Advancing critical care: joint combat casualty research team and joint theater trauma system. AACN Adv Crit Care 2010;21(3):260–76.

23. Frisch HM, Andersen RC, Mazurek MT, et al. The Military Extremity Trauma Amputation/Limb Salvage (METALS) study outcomes of amputation versus limb salvage following major lower-extremity trauma. J Bone Joint Surg Am 2013; 95(2):138–45.

24. Taylor BC, Hagel EM, Carlson KF, et al. Prevalence and costs of co-occurring traumatic brain injury with and without psychiatric disturbance and pain among Afghanistan and Iraq War veteran VA users. Med Care 2012;50(4):342–6.

25. Lew HL, Otis JD, Tun C, et al. Prevalence of chronic pain, posttraumatic stress disorder, and persistent post-concussive symptoms in OIF/OEF Veterans: polytrauma clinical triad. J Rehab Res Dev 2009;46(6):697.

26. Centers for Disease Control and Prevention (CDC). Vital signs: overdoses of prescription opioid pain relievers—United States, 1999–2008. MMWR Morb Mortal Wkly Rep 2011;60(43):1487–92.

27. Baliki NM, Petre B, Torbey S, et al. Corticostriatal functional connectivity predicts transition to chronic back pain. Nat Neurosci 2012;15:1117–9.

28. Ossipov MH, Morimura K, Porreca F. Descending pain modulation and chronification of pain. Curr Opin Support Palliat Care 2014;8(2):143–51.

29. Baliki MN, Huang L, Torbey S, et al. Brain white matter structural properties predict transition to chronic pain. Pain 2013;154(10):2160–8.

30. Hashmi JA, Baliki MN, Huang L, et al. Shape shifting pain: chronification of back pain shifts brain representation from nociceptive to emotional circuits. Brain 2013; 136(Pt 9):2751–68.

31. Gallagher RM. Management strategies for chronic pain. In: Krames ES, Peckham PH, Rezai AR, editors. Neuromodulation. New York: Academic Press; 2009. p. 313–32.

32. Akarian AV, Centeno MV, Kan L, et al. Role of adult hippocampal neurogenesis in persistent pain. Pain 2016;157:418–28.

33. Lieberman MD, Eisenberger NI. Pains and pleasures of social life. Science 2009; 323:890–1.

34. Gallagher RM. Rational integration of pharmacologic, behavioral, and rehabilitation strategies in the treatment of chronic pain. Am J Phys Med Rehabil 2005;84: S64–76.

35. Stojadinovic A, Auton A, Peoples GE, et al. Responding to challenges in modern combat casualty care: innovative use of advanced regional anesthesia. Pain Med 2006;7(4):330–8.

36. Polomano RC, Buckenmaier CC, Kwon KH. Effects of low-dose IV ketamine on peripheral and central pain from major limb injuries sustained in combat. Pain Med 2013;14(7):1088–100.

37. Castillo RC, MacKenzie EJ, Wegener ST, et al. Prevalence of chronic pain seven years following limb threatening lower extremity trauma. Pain 2006;124(3):321–9.

38. Buckenmaier CC III, Rupprecht C, McKnight G. Pain following battlefield injury and evacuation: a survey of 110 casualties from the wars in Iraq and Afghanistan. Pain Med 2009;10(8):1487–96.

39. Gallagher RM. Integrating medical and behavioral treatment in chronic pain management. Med Clin North Am 1999;83(5):823–49.

40. Lippe PM, Brock C, David J, et al. The first national pain medicine summit—final summary report. Pain Med 2010;11:1447–68.

41. Edlund MJ, Austen MA, Sullivan MD, et al. Patterns of opioid use for chronic non-cancer pain in the Veterans Health Administration from 2009 to 2011. Pain 2014; 155:2337–43.

42. Dobscha SK, Corson K, Perrin NA, et al. Collaborative care for chronic pain in primary care: a cluster-randomized trial. JAMA 2009;301(12):1242–52.

43. Westanmo A, Marshall P, Jones E, et al. Opioid dose reduction in a VA health care system—implementation of a primary care population-level initiative. Pain Med 2015;16:1019–26.

44. Frank JW, Carey EP, Fagan KM, et al. Evaluation of a telementoring intervention for pain management in the Veterans Health Administration. Pain Med 2015; 16(6):1090–100.

45. Gallagher RM. The pain medicine and primary care community rehabilitation model: monitored care for pain disorders in multiple settings. Clin J Pain 1999; 15(1):1–3.

46. Gallagher RM. Pain medicine and primary care: a community solution to pain as a public health problem. Med Clin North Am 1999;83(5):555–85.

47. Gallagher RM, Myers P. Referral delay in back pain patients on worker's compensation: costs and policy implications. Psychosomatics 1996;37(3):270–84.

48. Weiner DK, Fang M, Gentili A, et al. Deconstructing chronic low back pain in the older adult—step by step evidence and expert-based recommendations for evaluation and treatment: Part I: hip osteoarthritis. Pain Med 2015;16(5):886–97.

49. Lisi AJ, Breuer P, Gallagher RM, et al. Deconstructing chronic low back pain in the older adult–step by step evidence and expert-based recommendations for evaluation and treatment: part II: myofascial pain. Pain Med 2015;16(7):1282–9.

50. Fatemi G, Fang MA, Breuer P, et al. Deconstructing chronic low back pain in the older adult—step by step evidence and expert-based recommendations for evaluation and treatment: part III: fibromyalgia syndrome. Pain Med 2015;16(9): 1709–19.

51. Carley JA, Karp JF, Gentili A, et al. Deconstructing chronic low back pain in the older adult: step by step evidence and expert-based recommendations for evaluation and treatment: part IV: depression. Pain Med 2015;16(11):2098–108.

52. DiNapoli EA, Craine M, Dougherty P, et al. Deconstructing chronic low back pain in the older adult – step by step evidence and expert-based recommendations for evaluation and treatment: part V: maladaptive coping. Pain Med 2016;17(1): 64–73.

53. VHA DIRECTIVE 2009-053, Pain management. Available at: http://www1.va.gov/vhapublications/ViewPublication.asp?pub_ID=2781. Accessed November 10, 2015.

54. Army Task Force Report, 2010. Available at: http://www.regenesisbio.com/pdfs/journal/pain_management_task_force_report.pdf. Accessed November 10, 2015.

55. Defense and Veterans Center for Integrative Pain Management. Available at: http://www.dvcipm.org/. Accessed November 10, 2015.

56. Rosenberger P, Philip EJ, Lee A, et al. The VHA's National Pain Management Strategy: implementing the stepped care model. Fed Pract 2011;28(8):39–42.

57. Matthias MS, Miech EJ, Myers LJ, et al. An expanded view of self-management: patients' perceptions of education and support in an intervention for chronic musculoskeletal pain. Pain Med 2012;13(8):1018–28.

58. Wiedemer N, Harden P, Arndt R, et al. The opioid renewal clinic, a primary care, managed approach to opioid therapy in chronic pain patients at risk for substance abuse. Pain Med 2007;8(7):573–84.

59. Bair M. Overcoming fears, frustrations, and competing demands: an effective integration of pain medicine and primary care to treat complex pain patients. Pain Med 2007;8(7):544–5.

60. Tew J, Klaus J, Oslin DW. The Behavioral Health Laboratory: building a stronger foundation for the patient-centered medical home. Fam Syst Health 2010;28(2): 130–45.

61. Kerns RD, Sellinger J, Goodin BR. Psychological treatment of chronic pain. Annu Rev Clin Psychol 2011;7:411–34.

62. VA/DoD Clinical Practice guidelines: management of opioid therapy for pain. Available at: http://www.va.gov/PAINMANAGEMENT/docs/CPG_opioidtherapy_fulltext.pdf. Accessed November 10, 2015.

63. Kroenke K, Bair MJ, Damush TM, et al. Optimized antidepressant therapy and pain self-management in primary care patients with depression and musculoskeletal pain: a randomized controlled trial. JAMA 2009;301(20):2099–110.

64. Bair MJ, Ang D, Wu J, et al. Evaluation of Stepped Care for Chronic Pain (ESCAPE) in veterans of the Iraq and Afghanistan conflicts. A randomized clinical trial. JAMA Intern Med 2015;175:682–9.

65. Dubois M, Gallagher RM, Lippe P. Pain medicine position paper. Pain Med 2009; 10(6):972–1000.

66. Murphy L, Clark ME, Dubyak PJ, et al. Implementing step three: components and importance of tertiary pain care. Fed Pract 2012;29:S44–8.

67. Murphy JL, Clark ME, Banou E. Opioid cessation and multidimensional outcomes following interdisciplinary chronic pain treatment. J Pain 2013;29:1109–17.

68. Fishman SM, Young HM, Arwood EL. Core competencies for pain management: results of an interprofessional consensus summit. Pain Med 2013;14:971–81.

69. Tick H, Chauvin SW, Brown M, et al. Core competencies in integrative pain care for entry-level primary care physicians. Pain Med 2015;16(11):2090–7.

70. Ahles TA, Wasson JH, Seville JL, et al. A controlled trial of methods for managing pain in primary care patients with or without co-occurring psychosocial problems. Ann Fam Med 2006;4(4):341–50.

71. Pain Mini-residency. Available at: http://www.va.gov/PAINMANAGEMENT/For_Providers.asp. Accessed November 15, 2015.

72. Niemzow R. Battlefield acupuncture. Available at: http://www.isla-laser.org/wp-content/uploads/Niemtzow-Battlefield-Acupuncture.pdf. Accessed November 10, 2015.

73. Tiered Acupuncture Training Across Clinical Settings (ATACS): Battlefield acupuncture in DoD and VA. Available at: http://www.dvcipm.org/clinical-resources/battle-field-acupuncture. Accessed November 10, 2015.

74. VA-DoD Joint Pain Education and Training Project (JPEP). Available at: http://www.dvcipm.org/clinical-resources/joint-pain-education-project-jpep Accessed November 10, 2015.

75. Arora S, Kalishman S, Dion D, et al. Partnering urban academic medical centers and rural primary care clinicians to provide complex chronic disease care. Health Aff (Millwood) 2011;30(6):1176–84.

76. Opioid Safety Initiative (OSI). Available at: http://www.va.gov/PAINMANAGEMENT/Opioid_Safety_Initiative_OSI.asp. Accessed November 10, 2015.

77. Opioid Safety Initiative Toolkit. Available at: http://www.va.gov/PAINMANAGEMENT/Opioid_Safety_Initiative_Toolkit.asp. Accessed November 10, 2015.

78. Taking Opioids Responsibly. Available at: http://www.ethics.va.gov/docs/policy/Taking_Opioids_Responsibly_2013528.pdf. Accessed November 10, 2015.

79. Opioid therapy risk report. Available at: http://www.blogs.va.gov/VAntage/17721/va-accelerates-deployment-nationwide-opioid-therapy-tool/. Accessed November 10, 2015.

80. Academic Detailing. Available at: http://www.va.gov/PAINMANAGEMENT/docs/OSI_1_Toolkit_Pain_Educational_Guide.pdf. Accessed November 10, 2015.

81. Roberts GE, Adams R. Impact of introducing anticoagulation-related prescribing guidelines in a hospital setting using academic detailing. Ther Clin Risk Manag 2006;2(3):309–16.

82. Gallagher RM. Educating providers in opioid analgesia and risk management: what works. Keynote Address, REMS Panel, FDA, July 19, 2010. Available at: http://www.thci.org/Opioid/jun10docs/Gallagher.pdf. Accessed November 10, 2015.

83. Trafton J, Martine S, Michel M, et al. Evaluation of the acceptability and usability of a decision support system to encourage safe and effective use of opioid therapy for chronic, noncancer pain by primary care providers. Pain Med 2010;11(4):575–85.

84. Olivia E. Opioid Overdose Education and Naloxone Distribution (OEND): preventing and responding to an opioid overdose. Spotlight on pain management. 9/2/14. Available at: http://www.hsrd.research.va.gov/for_researchers/cyber_seminars/archives/video_archive.cfm?SessionID=868. Accessed November 10, 2015.

85. Eaton LH, Gordon DB, Doorenba AZ. The effect of a pain resource nurse training program on pain management knowledge. 2014 Western Institute of Nursing Annual Communicating Nursing Research Conference. Available at: http://www.researchgate.net/publication/268145156. Accessed November 18, 2015.

86. Kerns R, Dobscha S. Pain among veterans returning from deployment in Iraq and Afghanistan: update on the Veterans Health Administration Pain Research Program. Pain Med 2009;10(7):1161–4.

87. Kerns R, Heapy A. Advances in pain management for veterans: current status of research and future directions. In: Kerns R, Heapy A, editors. Transforming pain care in the Veterans Health Administration: bridges from theory and research to practice and policy. Special issue, JRRD 2015, in press. Available at: http://www.rehab.research.va.gov/jour/2014/512/pdf/callforpapers512.pdf. Accessed November 17, 2015.

88. Gallagher RM. The pain research working group and pain care in the VHA. In: Kerns R, Heapy A, editors. Transforming pain care in the Veterans Health

Administration: bridges from theory and research to practice and policy. Special issue, JRRD 2015, in press. Available at: http://www.rehab.research.va.gov/jour/2014/512/pdf/callforpapers512.pdf. Accessed November 17, 2015.

89. Sturgeon JA, Darnall BD, Kao MC, et al. Physical and psychological correlates of fatigue and physical function: a Collaborative Health Outcomes Information Registry (CHOIR) study. J Pain 2015;16(3):291–8.

90. Pain Assessment Screening Tool and Outcomes Registry (PASTOR). Defense and Veterans Center for Integrated Pain Management. Available at: http://www.dvcipm.org/clinical-resources/pain-assessment-screening-tool-and-outcomes-registry-pastor. Accessed November 10, 2015.

91. The Interagency Pain Research Coordinating Committee. The National Pain Strategy: a comprehensive population health level strategy for pain. Available at: http://iprcc.nih.gov/National_Pain_Strategy/NPS_Main.htm. Accessed November 17, 2015.

Assessing and Managing Sleep Disturbance in Patients with Chronic Pain

Martin D. Cheatle, PhD[a,b,*], Simmie Foster, MD, PhD[c],
Aaron Pinkett, BS[a], Matthew Lesneski, MD[d], David Qu, MD[e],
Lara Dhingra, PhD[f]

KEYWORDS

- Chronic pain • Insomnia • Cognitive behavior therapy • Sleep-disordered breathing
- Pharmacotherapy

KEY POINTS

- Sleep disturbance is common in patients with chronic pain (CP).
- Sleep and pain are bidirectional; pain can interfere with sleep and sleep disturbance can exacerbate pain.
- The presence of sleep-disordered breathing, including obstructive sleep apnea and central sleep apnea, increases the risk of significant harm associated with the use of opioids and other centrally sedating medications.
- Cognitive behavior therapy (CBT) has the potential to improve both pain and sleep quality.
- There are several pharmacologic agents used to improve sleep disturbance in the CP population.

Conflicts of Interest: None of the authors has any conflicts of interest related to the material in this article.

[a] Department of Psychiatry, Center for Studies of Addiction, Perelman School of Medicine, University of Pennsylvania, 3535 Market Street, 4th Floor, Philadelphia, PA 19104, USA; [b] Department of Psychiatry, Behavioral Medicine Center, Reading Health System, 560 Van Reed Road, Suite 204, Wyomissing, PA 19610, USA; [c] Kirby Center for Neurobiology, 3 Blackfan Circle, CLS 12-260, Boston, MA 02115, USA; [d] RA Pain Services, 1500 Midatlantic Drive Suite 102, Mount Laurel, NJ 0854, USA; [e] Highpoint Pain and Rehabilitation Physicians P.C., 700 Horizon Circle Suite 206, Chalfont, PA 18914, USA; [f] MJHS Institute for Innovation in Palliative Care, 39 Broadway, 3rd Floor, New York, NY 10006, USA
* Corresponding author. Center for Studies of Addiction, Perelman School of Medicine, University of Pennsylvania, 3535 Market Street, 4th Floor, Philadelphia, PA 19104.
E-mail address: cheatle@mail.med.upenn.edu

Anesthesiology Clin 34 (2016) 379–393
http://dx.doi.org/10.1016/j.anclin.2016.01.007
1932-2275/16/$ – see front matter © 2016 Elsevier Inc. All rights reserved.

INTRODUCTION

Patients with CP often present to clinicians with numerous medical and psychological comorbidities, including mood and anxiety disorders, secondary medical problems related to inactivity and weight gain, and sleep disturbance. Insomnia can be generally defined as the inability to acquire adequate sleep to feel rested in the morning. Insomnia can be due to difficulties initiating or maintaining sleep or both. Chronic insomnia (occurring at least 3 times per week for at least 3 months) usually leads to daytime consequences, such as fatigue, reduced mental acuity, and so forth.

It has been estimated that the prevalence of sleep disturbance in patients with CP ranges between 50% and 80%.[1–5] For example, Tang and colleagues[1] evaluated 70 patients with chronic back pain and compared them to 70 gender-matched and age-matched pain-free control patients, measuring sleep disturbance, pain, and a variety of psychological variables, including health status anxiety and depression. Results indicated that 53% of the patients with CP demonstrated evidence of clinical insomnia, with only 3% of the pain-free controls meeting criteria for insomnia. Furthermore, insomnia severity was positively associated with pain intensity, sensory pain ratings, affective pain ratings, general anxiety, general depression, and health anxiety. Affective pain ratings and health status anxiety were the best predictors of insomnia severity, which suggests that emotional distress is strongly linked to sleep disturbance. In another study by McCracken and colleagues,[2] 159 patients undergoing evaluation at a pain management center were assessed for history of sleep disturbance. In this cohort, 79% met criteria for significant insomnia based on self-reported symptoms.

There is persuasive evidence to support the hypothesis that the association between pain and sleep are bidirectional in nature.[6,7] Sivertsen and colleagues[7] collected data on CP and sleep and assessed experimental pain sensitivity via cold pressor testing in 10,412 adults in Norway. The results of this study revealed that insomnia frequency and severity, sleep-onset problems, and sleep efficiency were positively associated with pain sensitivity. Results also revealed that pain tolerance was reduced further in a synergistic fashion in subjects who reported both CP and insomnia. Clinical studies have proved that CP patients who reported sleep disturbance also note increased pain, more fatigue, poor mood, and generally higher levels of stress and disability.[8,9] Experimental studies in healthy controls demonstrate that sleep deprivation or disruption leads to an increase in pain via an increase in the release of proinflammatory cytokines[10] and a decrease in pain tolerance.[11] There has also been some speculation that pain, sleep, and depression share underlying neurobiological mechanisms.[12]

Despite the burgeoning evidence for the bidirectional association between pain and sleep and the deleterious effects of sleep deprivation on mood, pain sensitivity, and disability, addressing sleep disturbance in patients with CP is often overlooked in the clinical encounter due to the many competing concerns. The aim of this article is to provide clinicians with a basic understanding of assessing sleep disturbance and the use of nonpharmacologic and pharmacologic treatment strategies to improve sleep quality in patients with CP. This article does not include a discussion of other sleep disorders, in particular, sleep-disordered breathing (obstructive sleep apnea and central sleep apnea). It is critical to assess and monitor obstructive sleep apnea and central sleep apnea in patients considered for opioid therapy or who are receiving opioids, because a significant percentage of patients on opioid therapy has sleep-disordered breathing. A recently published article by Cheatle and Webster[13] specifically addresses the topic of sleep-disordered breathing and opioids in patients with CP.

ASSESSMENT OF SLEEP DISTURBANCE

Polysomnography (PSG) and self-report measures of sleep disturbance are standard approaches used in insomnia research. More recently, actigraphy has been used as an objective measure of sleep quality in sleep research. There are also several commercially available activity-sleep monitors that can be used clinically in assessing and monitoring sleep duration. Self-report questionnaires are more commonly used because they

1. Are inexpensive
2. Are the primary assessment tool used by clinicians treating insomnia
3. Standardize methods across research studies given the lack of a biomarker for insomnia and a universally accepted definition of insomnia[14]

The selection of a self-report measure depends on a clinician's goals. These goals may vary from screening and diagnosis to monitoring of previously identified sleep disturbances to evaluating the efficacy of treatment interventions. There are several sleep assessment scales that evaluate multiple dimensions of sleep, including sleep quality, sleep onset, postsleep evaluation, and generic outcomes. Of these, sleep quality and postsleep evaluation measures are the most commonly used. Examples of various sleep instruments are outlined in **Table 1**.[15–20] Moul and colleagues[14] also provide a comprehensive review of the different sleep scales.

Each measure has varying degrees of utility depending on the nature of the sleep disturbance, the level of severity, and the specific characteristics of sleep a

Table 1
Self-report measures for assessment of insomnia

Domain	Scale	Time Frame	No. of Items	Comments
Postsleep evaluation	Wolff's Morning Questions[14]	Today	8	Yes/no questions detailing morning restedness, presence of bedpartner, etc.
Postsleep evaluation	Kryger's Subjective Measurements[15]	Today	9	Mixed format questions detailing sleep onset, sleep latency, etc.
Postsleep evaluation	Morning Sleep Questionnaire[16]	Today	4	Mixed format questions evaluating sleep goodness and other factors
Sleep quality	Pittsburgh Sleep Quality Index[17]	Past month	24	Mixed format questions and household-related questions that use an algorithm to score sleep disturbance
Sleep quality	Sleep Questionnaire[18]	Indefinite	59	Questions use Likert-type scale responses ranging from sleep depth to dream recall/vividness
Sleep quality	Sleep Disturbance Questionnaire[19]	Indefinite	12	Questions use Likert-type scale responses that assess mental anxiety and physical tension

Data from Refs.[14–19]

clinician seeks to assess. It is important to select a sleep instrument that fits the dynamics of the clinical setting, such as time constraints, patient burden, and staff resources.

NONPHARMACOLOGIC INTERVENTIONS
Cognitive Behavior Therapy for Pain and Sleep

Medications are commonly used to manage both pain and insomnia; however, the use of medications can result in adverse effects, dependence, and poor treatment efficacy. The use of nonpharmacologic approaches for pain and insomnia may mitigate these negative effects, but clinicians seldom implement psychological strategies. Evidence-based CBT approaches for pain (CBT-P) and for insomnia (CBT-I) are well developed, efficacious, and cost effective and may improve clinical outcomes and treatment response for different subpopulations with varied pain conditions. Many clinicians lack training in the effective use of CBT techniques, however, or there is poor access to these services.

Cognitive behavior therapy for pain

A variety of psychological and behavioral strategies are effective for CP management, including CBT, acceptance and commitment therapy, mindfulness-based stress reduction, progressive muscle relaxation training, motivational interviewing, and goal setting to increase behavioral activation.[21–23] CBT may incorporate any of these specific components. CBT techniques usually involve the identification of maladaptive or dysfunctional thoughts and behaviors that may worsen patient adjustment to CP and disability. The evaluation and modification of negative thought patterns and their substitution with more rational cognitions can reframe patients' interpretations that contribute to feelings of suffering, demoralization, and helplessness. CBT may assist patients in developing and implementing specific strategies, such as progressive muscle relaxation train, activity pacing, distraction techniques, and positive self-talk, to help them cope with negative affect caused by pain and disability.

CBT-P has been shown highly effective at reducing patient distress in a variety of pain disorders.[24–27] It might be expected that improved pain would translate into improved sleep for patients. It is difficult, however, to make this conclusion because few studies evaluating the efficacy of CBT-P in a CP population have examined sleep. Although the data are inconclusive, the few studies that included sleep measures suggested minimal improvement in sleep after CBT-P.[28,29] Based on this observation, CP patients suffering from insomnia may achieve the most improvement in sleep from interventions that specifically target sleep disturbance.

Cognitive behavior therapy for insomnia

In studies of patients with chronic primary insomnia, CBT-I has been shown equally effective or even superior to pharmacotherapy in multiple outcomes. Sivertsen and colleagues[30] compared CBT-I to standard therapy with eszopiclone and found that the CBT-I treatment group had increased time spent in slow-wave restorative sleep and improved sleep efficiency (proportion of time spent in bed actually sleeping).

A course of CBT-I typically consists of

- Psychoeducation about sleep and insomnia
- Stimulus control
- Sleep restriction
- Sleep hygiene
- Relaxation training
- Cognitive therapy

Stimulus control strengthens a patient's association of the bed with rapid-onset sleep, by teaching the patient to limit the use of bed to sex and sleep, avoid daytime naps, maintain a regular sleep/wake time, go to bed only when sleepy, and get out of bed if not asleep within 15 to 20 minutes. Sleep restriction limits the amount of time a patient spends in bed to the actual time asleep, so, for example, if a patient spends 8 hours in bed but only 4 hours total asleep, the patient is instructed to spend only 4 hours in bed. This leads initially to a mild sleep deprivation, which increases the patient's drive to sleep and leads to more consolidated, restful sleep and greater sleep efficiency. Over time, as sleep efficiency improves, the patient gradually increases time in bed. Sleep hygiene increases patients' awareness of behavioral and environmental factors that have an impact on sleep, such as how caffeine, alcohol, periods of intense exercise, bright lights, and use of electronic devices before bed may be detrimental to sleep, as well as education on the benefits of a restful bedroom environment. Relaxation training reduces cognitive and physical tension close to bedtime and involves techniques, such as hypnosis, meditation, and guided imagery. Cognitive therapy helps patients explore how beliefs and attitudes toward sleep affect sleep behaviors. Patients learn to identify maladaptive or distorted thoughts and replace them with more adaptive substitutes, thereby helping to alleviate worrying or rumination about insomnia.

CBT-I has been shown in several studies to improve sleep in patients with CP. For example, Jungquist and colleagues,[31] in a study of 28 patients with chronic back and neck pain, found that those patients who received CBT-I had significantly improved sleep and maintained improvements in total sleep time at 6 months post-treatment completion, despite the persistence of moderate to severe pain.

Combined treatment of pain and sleep

Given the effectiveness of CBT-I and of CBT-P, there has been growing interest in the feasibility of combining CBT-I with CBT-P. In a small pilot study of 20 patients with CP, Tang and colleagues[32] found that a hybrid CBT-I/CBT-P intervention was associated with greater improvement in sleep at post-treatment. Although pain intensity did not change, the hybrid group reported greater reductions in pain interference, fatigue, and depression than the controls, and overall changes were clinically significant and durable at 1-month and 6-month follow-ups. Thus current evidence suggests that CBT is an important treatment that should be used in the treatment of insomnia in CP patients.

PHARMACOTHERAPY

For many patients with CP, uncontrolled pain precipitates sleep and mood disturbance, so naturally clinicians often first focus exclusively on treating pain.[33] Due to the reciprocal relationship between pain and sleep, however, it is important to concurrently treat sleep disorders; pharmacologic treatments aimed at improvements in sleep have been shown to decrease pain intensity.[34,35] Given the complex presentation of patients with CP and sleep disturbance, clinicians usually tailor pharmacologic therapy for insomnia based on a patients pain pathophysiology and comorbid conditions. The most commonly used medications for insomnia are reviewed and their role for patients with CP and sleep disturbance highlighted. An overview of pharmacologic sleep agents, dosing, and adverse effects is in **Table 2**.

Opioid Analgesics

Several studies have shown that opioid medications may improve subjective quality of sleep; for example, 1 study in patients with osteoarthritis found that extended-release

Table 2
Pharmacologic sleep agents, dosing, and adverse effects

Agent	Dose	Adverse Effects	Comments
Amitriptyline	10–100 mg	Orthostatic hypotension, daytime sedation, anticholinergic effects, cardiac conduction abnormality, sexual dysfunction, weight gain	Used for neuropathic pain, tension headaches, and fibromyalgia
Doxepin	3–6 mg proprietary, 10–100 mg generic	Minimal anticholinergic side effects at hypnotic doses	FDA approved for insomnia
Mirtazapine	7.5–30 mg	Increased appetite, weight gain, anticholinergic effects	Excellent for patients with poor appetite, mood and sleep disturbance
Trazodone	25–100 mg	Dizziness, anticholinergic effects, daytime sedation, priapism, neuropathic pain	May be helpful in diabetic neuropathy and fibromyalgia
Temazepam	15–50 mg	Sedation, fatigue, depression, dizziness, ataxia, confusion	FDA approved for insomnia; no evidence for long-term use
Clonazepam	0.5–3 mg	Sedation, fatigue, depression, dizziness, ataxia, confusion	Used for restless leg syndrome, anxiety, muscle spasm, anticonvulsant activity. May be beneficial for patients with neuropathic pain; no evidence or long-term use for sleep
Zolpidem	5–10 mg (immediate release) 6.25–12.5 mg (extended release)	Aberrant sleep-related behaviors	Most prescribed hypnotic
Zaleplon	5–20 mg	—	Shortest active BzRA; useful for patients with nocturnal awakenings
Eszopiclone	1–03 mg	Unpleasant taste, sedation, dizziness	Well tolerated; may boost antidepressant and anxiolytic efficacy
Melatonin	0.5–3 mg	—	Well tolerated; over-the-counter no FDA approval; useful for shift workers/delayed sleep phase

(*continued on next page*)

Agent	Dose	Adverse Effects	Comments
Ramelteon	8 mg	—	FDA approved; few adverse effects other than sedation, main effect on sleep latency
Quetiapine	25–50 mg	Dry mouth, weight gain, metabolic syndromes, orthostatic hypotension rare dystonias	Effective in anxiety disorders
Gabapentin	100–900 mg	Dizziness, ataxia, fatigue, weight gain, lower extremity swelling	Used for neuropathic pain, fibromyalgia with comorbid sleep disturbance
Diphenhydramine	25–50 mg	Anticholinergic side effects	Caution with elderly, no literature to support chronic use, no evidence for pain control

Table 2
(continued)

morphine sulfate was associated with improvements in objective sleep measures of PSG, including sleep efficiency.[36] In contrast, there have also been studies that demonstrate that opioids can inhibit both rapid eye movement and non–rapid eye movement sleep, contributing to an exacerbation of pain.[37,38] There is also compelling evidence that long-term use of opioid analgesics may lead to adverse effects, including sleep-disordered breathing, opioid-induced hyperalgesia, tolerance, and dependence in populations at risk.[39] Therefore, although opioids may be effective in carefully selected patients for the treatment of pain, opioids should never be used to treat insomnia.

Benzodiazepine Receptor Agonists

Benzodiazepine receptor agonists (BzRAS) include benzodiazepines (eg, temazepam and triazolam) and the newer class of nonbenzodiazepine drugs (eg, zolpidem and eszopiclone). This class of drugs binds to γ-aminobutyric acid (GABA)-A receptors and induces sedative/hypnotic, amnestic, anxiolytic, muscle relaxant, and anticonvulsant effects.[40,41] Many short-term clinical trials show that BzRAs improve sleep quality, sleep latency, wakefulness after sleep onset, and total sleep time.[40] Most benzodiazepines (excluding triazolam) have intermediate to long half-lives and, therefore, may help patients fall asleep and stay asleep.

Food and Drug Administration (FDA)-approved benzodiazepines for insomnia include temazepam, triazolam, estazolam, quazepam, and flurazepam.[42] Lorazepam, alprazolam, and clonazepam are anxiolytics that are often used off-label for sleep. For patients with CP, short-term use of benzodiazepines may be useful in improving muscle tension, anxiety, and neuropathic pain as well as sleep.[43,44] One early study found, however, that with long-term use (>1 year), pain patients using benzodiazepines reported no significant clinical improvements in sleep.[45]

Although the benzodiazepines may work well in short-term efficacy trials, few data are available on long-term use, and there are many documented adverse effects. In the elderly, standard doses may lead to ataxia and psychomotor impairment, which may increase the risk of falls and hip fractures.[46] All BzRAs can cause cognitive impairment and decreased attention, specifically anterograde amnesia.[47] Long-term use of benzodiazepines may increase depressive symptomatology, with cognitive and psychomotor slowing.[45] In addition, abruptly stopping the drug may lead to rebound insomnia and seizures. There is also a concern of tolerance and dependence, especially in patients with a history of sedative or alcohol abuse.[48]

Care should be taken to not use more than 1 benzodiazepine at once (for example, temazepam for sleep and clonazepam for muscle relaxation), because many drugs in this class have active metabolites that can combine and lead to delayed sedation.[40] Also, the use of benzodiazepines in combination with opioids presents increased risk of harm to patients, especially those patients with sleep-disordered breathing. In addition, combining opioids with benzodiazepines should be avoided in patients with depression, especially in those patients with suicidal ideation.

Nonbenzodiazepine Benzodiazepine Receptor Agonists

The nonbenzodiazepine BzRAs (NBzRAs), zolpidem, zaleplon, and eszopiclone, are the newest class of FDA-approved hypnotics used for insomnia. They universally improve sleep latency and have the potential for fewer daytime side effects give their shorter half-lives and receptor binding profile. Long-term efficacy trials have supported their use.[49,50]

Zolpidem is currently the most widely prescribed drug for insomnia. In contrast to the benzodiazepines, 1 double-blind, placebo-controlled study showed that nightly use of zolpidem remained effective after 8 months of nightly use with no evidence of tolerance or rebound effects.[50]

Eszopiclone was approved by the FDA for the treatment of insomnia with no short-term restrictions on use. Similar to zolpidem, studies suggest that eszopiclone is effective for 6 to 12 months of long-term use.[51] In addition, eszopiclone augments the effects of antidepressants and anxiolytics in patients who have insomnia and co-morbid depression or anxiety.[49]

The use of both zolpidem and eszopiclone is associated with improved sleep and quality of life in fibromyalgia and rheumatoid arthritis patients.[44,52,53] In terms of safety, similar to triazolam, zolpidem and zaleplon are associated with sleep-related behaviors, including sleep eating, sleep walking, and sleep driving.[40] For zolpidem, recent data on cognitive function and drug blood levels have prompted the FDA to lower the recommended daily dose for women.[40] In contrast to studies of typical benzodiazepines, recent studies of zolpidem, zaleplon, and eszoplicone have not noted tolerance or discontinuation effects. Although there are limited and conflicting data on the potential risk of this class of medications on sleep-disordered breathing[54] there is some evidence that NBzRAS have contributed to deaths, typically in combination with other central nervous system depressants, including opioids.[55] Clinicians should consider the potential added risk of prescribing NBzRAS to patients with CP receiving opioids and alternatively use medications for insomnia with a lower risk profile.

Antidepressants

Sedative antidepressants, such as tricyclic antidepressants (TCAs), mirtazapine, and trazodone, are useful in treating CP patients with insomnia by helping to relieve

1. Insomnia
2. Depressive symptoms that likely enhance pain perception
3. The pain condition itself[33]

TCAs (amitriptyline, nortriptyline, desipramine, clomipramine, imipramine, trimipramine, and doxepin) have proserotonergic, noradrenergic, dopaminergic, and sodium-channel blocking effects that may account for their efficacy in pain and depression, along with anticholinergic and antihistaminic effects that lead to sedation. At standard doses, all TCAs have shown equal efficacy in treating neuropathic pain; however, they are not all equal in promoting sleep.[56,57] For example, desipramine and imipramine are less sedating and may disrupt sleep.[58,59] Amitriptyline, nortriptyline, trimipramine, and doxepin, on the other hand, may decrease sleep latency, increase sleep efficiency, and increase total sleep time.[56,60]

Amitriptyline is probably the best studied TCA for improving sleep in patients with comorbid pain, especially headache, fibromyalgia, and neuropathic pain.[61–63] It may be poorly tolerated, however, due to anticholinergic side effects. Nortriptyline, a metabolite of amitriptyline, may cause less sedation but may also have fewer side effects, including less daytime drowsiness.[64]

Doxepin, the only TCA approved by the FDA for the treatment of insomnia, has a hypnotic dose of 1 mg to 6 mg as opposed to 150 mg to 300 mg when used as an antidepressant. At the lower doses, doxepin is selective for histamine type 1 receptors, which may explain its sedative effects without typical anticholinergic adverse effects. Safety and efficacy studies revealed reduced wakefulness after sleep onset, increased sleep efficiency, and total sleep time without next-day sedation or anticholinergic effects.[65] At these doses, doxepin has not been formally studied for an analgesic or antidepressant effect, although it may be titrated as tolerated to improve pain syndromes.[41]

Adverse effects of TCAs, due to anti–α-adrenergic and anticholinergic effects, include orthostatic hypotension, dry mouth and eyes, constipation, and cardiac conduction delays. In addition, TCAs may prolong the QT interval, leading to increased risk for serious cardiac arrhythmias. Risks of cardiac-related adverse effects, including orthostatic hypotension, increase with increased age. The blood levels of TCAs can be increased by the concurrent use of several medications, including selective serotonin reuptake inhibitors. Because the risk for serious adverse events is increased with increased TCA blood levels, care must be taken to carefully consider concurrent medications and make appropriate dose adjustments when indicated. Clinicians must also be cautious when prescribing TCAs to depressed and suicidal patients, because they are extremely lethal in overdose (lethality may occur with as little as 1 g).[66]

Trazodone is an antagonist of serotonin type 2, histamine, and α_1-adrenergic receptors, and mildly inhibits serotonin reuptake. Similar to the other antidepressants, trazodone exerts most of its hypnotic effects at low doses and has antidepressant effects at higher doses. Several studies show that trazodone improves sleep in the elderly, depressed patients, and patients with anxiety disorders and posttraumatic stress disorder.[67] Trazodone has also been studied in patients with various pain syndromes, including fibromyalgia and diabetic neuropathy, where it was associated with both improved pain and sleep quality.[68,69] There is also some evidence for adjunctive effects when used with pregabalin for CP patients.[67] There are concerns about tolerance with this drug, however; in 1 study trazodone was shown as effective as zolpidem on sleep latency and total sleep time but only during the first 2 weeks of therapy.[70] Side effects include next-day drowsiness, rebound insomnia, orthostatic hypotension, dry mouth, and, rarely, priapism.

Mirtazapine is an antidepressant with sedating qualities due to the antagonism of type 1 histaminergic and serotonin type 2 receptors. At doses of 15 mg to 30 mg, it improves sleep latency, total sleep time, and sleep efficiency and decreases frequency of night awakenings.[56] It has been shown to improve sleep, pain, appetite, and mood in cancer patients.[71] In addition, several studies have suggested that mirtazapine is useful for the treatment of pain caused by recurrent headache and postherpetic neuralgia.[72–74]

Selective serotonin reuptake inhibitors and serotonin-norepinephrine reuptake inhibitors (SNRIs), although effective for depression and pain, have been shown to disrupt and fragment sleep.[60] Duloxetine, an SNRI, is often used to treat neuropathic pain and comorbid mood but has been shown to decrease sleep efficiency.[33,61] Dosing of the SNRI during the day and avoiding SNRI use in the evening hours may help to mitigate this adverse effect.

Antipsychotics

Two of the newer atypical antipsychotic medications, quetiapine and olanzapine, are used off-label for the treatment of insomnia. Self-reported outcomes and PSG data suggest efficacy in increasing total sleep time and slow wave restorative sleep and in decreasing sleep latency.[64,75] At low doses, quetiapine primarily has antihistiminergic properties and is weakly proserotonergic. It has been shown to decrease anxiety and enhance the effects of antidepressant medication.[64] In addition, several case reports and open-label studies show that quetiapine and olanzapine have analgesic properties, especially for fibromyalgia and migraine disorders.[75,76] These medications may cause significant weight gain (olanzapine more so than quetiapine), however. Cardiac conduction abnormalities (such as prolonged QT interval) should be monitored in patients using these drugs. In addition, there is a small risk of movement disorders, such as akathisia and tardive dyskinesia. If atypical antipsychotics are considered, it is advisable to do so in consultation with a psychiatrist.

Anticonvulsants

Gabapentin and pregabalin are GABA analogs often used to treat CP conditions with comorbid insomnia.[33] Across multiple studies of patients with neuropathic pain and fibromyalgia, self-reported sleep outcomes suggest positive effects on sleep latency and wakefulness after sleep onset as well as increased deep sleep.[33,77,78] Both drugs also have adjunctive effects on depression and anxiety.[79] A recent study showed that pregabalin was more effective in improving sleep among patients with diabetic neuropathy compared with amitriptyline.[61] Common adverse effects include dizziness, next-day sedation, gastrointestinal symptoms, and peripheral edema.

Over-the-Counter Medications

Melatonin receptor agonists include the natural ligand melatonin as well as nonmelatonin drugs such as ramelteon. Melatonin has been shown to induce sleep by attenuating the wake-promoting impulses in the suprachiasmatic nucleus of the hypothalamus. Melatonin is available over the counter and is not FDA approved. In 2005, the FDA approved ramelteon, a melatonin receptor agonist, for the treatment of sleep-onset insomnia. Both melatonin and ramelteon have mild efficacy for reducing sleep latency, especially in patients who have delayed sleep phases (sleep and wake times shifted later).[80] This population frequently includes older adults and shift workers. There is some evidence that melatonin may have analgesic effects in patients with fibromyalgia, irritable bowel syndrome, and migraine disorders.[81]

Most other over-the-counter sleep agents contain first-generation antihistamines, such as diphenhydramine and doxylamine, which also have anticholinergic effects. Diphenhydramine is the most commonly used nonprescription sleep aid. Patients, however, may quickly develop tolerance. To date there are no controlled trials that demonstrate the efficacy of diphenhydramine for greater than 3 weeks in the treatment of insomnia. Antihistamines can cause next-day sedation and impair cognitive function and should be used with caution in the elderly.

SUMMARY

Sleep disturbance commonly occurs in patients with CP and can cause additional distress and fatigue and may exacerbate pain. There is persuasive evidence that pain and sleep have a bidirectional relationship; pain can cause sleep disturbance and sleep disturbance can increase pain. Typically, sleep disturbance is not systematically evaluated, treated, and monitored in busy pain care settings. There are multiple evidenced-based nonpharmacologic and pharmacologic approaches that can significantly improve both sleep disturbance and co-occurring pain, and some may reduce the use of opioids in specific patients on long-term opioid therapy. The assessment of the multiple dimensions of sleep and basic treatment strategies should be incorporated into the routine care of patients with CP and included in pain education and training for professionals.

REFERENCES

1. Tang NK, Wright KJ, Salkovskis PM. Prevalence and correlates of clinical insomnia co-occurring with chronic back pain. J Sleep Res 2007;16(1):85–95.
2. McCracken LM, Williams JL, Tang NK. Psychological flexibility may reduce insomnia in persons with chronic pain: a preliminary retrospective study. Pain Med 2011;12(6):904–12.
3. Allen KD, Renner JB, DeVellis B, et al. Osteoarthritis and sleep: the Johnston County Osteoarthritis Project. J Rheumatol 2008;35:1102–7.
4. Artner J, Cakir B, Spiekermann JA, et al. Prevalence of sleep deprivation in patients with chronic neck and back pain: a retrospective evaluation of 1016 patients. J Pain Res 2013;6:1–6.
5. Alsaadi SM, McAuley JH, Hush JM, et al. Prevalence of sleep disturbance in patients with low back pain. Eur Spine J 2011;20(5):737–43.
6. Koffel E, Kroenke K, Bair MJ, et al. The bidirectional relationship between sleep complaints and pain: analysis of data from a randomized trial. Health Psychol 2016;35(1):41–9.
7. Sivertsen B, Lallukka T, Petrie KJ, et al. Sleep and pain sensitivity in adults. Pain 2015;156(8):1433–9.
8. Haythornthwaite JA, Hegel MT, Kerns RD. Development of a sleep diary for chronic pain patients. J Pain Symptom Manage 1991;6(2):65–72.
9. Chiu YH, Silman AJ, Macfarlane GJ, et al. Poor sleep and depression are independently associated with a reduced pain threshold. Results of a population based study. Pain 2005;115(3):316–21.
10. Moldofsky H, Lue FA, Eisen J, et al. The relationship of interleukin-1 and immune functions to sleep in humans. Psychosom Med 1986;48(5):309–18.
11. Onen SH, Alloui A, Gross A, et al. The effects of total sleep deprivation, selective sleep interruption and sleep recovery on pain tolerance thresholds in healthy subjects. J Sleep Res 2001;10(1):35–42.
12. Boakye PA, Olechowski C, Rashiq S, et al. A critical review of neurobiological factors involved in the interactions between chronic pain, depression, and sleep disruption. Clin J Pain 2015. [Epub ahead of print].
13. Cheatle MD, Webster LR. Opioid therapy and sleep disorders: risks and mitigation strategies. Pain Med 2015;16(Suppl 1):S22–6.

14. Moul DE, Hall M, Pilkonis PA, et al. Self-report measures of insomnia in adults: rationales, choices, and needs. Sleep Med Rev 2004;8(3):177–98.

15. Wolff BB. Evaluation of hypnotics in outpatients with insomnia using a questionnaire and a self-rating technique. Clin Pharmacol Ther 1974;15(2):130–40.

16. Kryger MH, Steljes D, Pouliot Z, et al. Subjective versus objective evaluation of hypnotic efficacy: experience with zolpidem. Sleep 1991;14(5):399–407.

17. Mendelson WB, Maczaj M. Effects of triazolam on the perception of wakefulness in insomniacs. Ann Clin Psychiatry 1990;2:211–5.

18. Buysse DJ, Reynolds CF 3rd, Monk TH, et al. The Pittsburgh Sleep Quality Index: a new instrument for psychiatric practice and research. Psychiatry Res 1989; 28(2):193–213.

19. Domino G, Blair G, Bridges A. Subjective assessment of sleep by Sleep Questionnaire. Percept Mot Skills 1984;59(1):163–70.

20. Espie CA, Brooks DN, Lindsay WR. An evaluation of tailored psychological treatment of insomnia. J Behav Ther Exp Psychiatry 1989;20(2):143–53.

21. McCracken LM, Turk TC. Behavioral and cognitive-behavioral treatment for chronic pain: outcome, predictors of outcome, and treatment process. Spine (Phila Pa 1976) 2002;27(22):2564.

22. McCracken LM, Eccleston C, Vowles KE. Acceptance-based treatment for persons with complex, long standing chronic pain: a preliminary analysis of treatment outcome in comparison to a waiting phase. Behav Res Ther 2005;43: 1335–46.

23. Williams AC, Eccleston C, Morley S. Psychological therapies for the management of chronic pain (excluding headache) in adults. Cochrane Database Syst Rev 2012;(11):CD007407.

24. Keefe FJ, Caldwell DS. Cognitive behavioral control of arthritis pain. Med Clin North Am 1997;81:277–90.

25. Glombiewski JA, Hartwich-Tersek J, Rief W. Two psychological interventions are effective in severely disabled, chronic back pain patients: a randomized controlled trial. Int J Behav Med 2010;17(2):97–107.

26. Turner JA, Manci L, Aaron LA. Short- and long-term efficacy of brief cognitive-behavioral therapy for patients with chronic tempromandibular disorder pain: a randomized, controlled trial. Pain 2006;121(3):181–94.

27. Thieme K, Flor H, Turk D. Psychological pain treatment in fibromyalgia syndrome: efficacy of operant behavioral and cognitive behavioral treatments. Arthritis Res Ther 2006;8(4):R121.

28. Becker N, Sjøgren P, Bech P, et al. Treatment outcome of chronic non-malignant pain patients managed in a Danish multidisciplinary pain centre compared to general practice: a randomized controlled trial. Pain 2000;84(2–3):203–11.

29. Tang NK. Cognitive-behavioral therapy for sleep abnormalities of chronic pain patients. Curr Rheumatol Rep 2009;11(6):451–60.

30. Sivertsen B, Omvik S, Pallesen S, et al. Cognitive behavioral therapy vs zopiclone for treatment of chronic primary insomnia in older adults: a randomized controlled trial. JAMA 2006;295(24):2851–8.

31. Jungquist CR, Tra Y, Smith MT, et al. The durability of cognitive behavioral therapy for insomnia in patients with chronic pain. Sleep Disord 2012;2012:679648.

32. Tang NK, Goodchild CE, Salkovskis PM. Hybrid cognitive-behavior therapy for individuals with insomnia and chronic pain: a pilot randomized controlled trial. Behav Res Ther 2012;50(12):814–21.

33. Argoff C. The coexistence of neuropathic pain, sleep, and psychiatric disorders: a novel treatment approach. Clin J Pain 2007;23:15–22.

34. Roehrs T, Roth T. Sleep and pain: interaction of two vital functions. Semin Neurol 2005;25(1):106–16.
35. Wilson KG, Eriksson MY, D'Eon JL, et al. Major depression and insomnia in chronic pain. Clin J Pain 2002;18:77–83.
36. Rosenthal M, Moore P, Groves E, et al. Sleep improves when patients with chronic OA pain are managed with morning dosing of once a day extended-release morphine sulfate (AVINZA): findings from a pilot study. J Opioid Manag 2007; 3(3):145–54.
37. Shaw IR, Lavigne G, Mayer P, et al. Acute intravenous administration of morphine perturbs sleep architecture in healthy pain-free young adults: a preliminary study. Sleep 2005;28(6):677–82.
38. Rosenberg J. Sleep disturbances after non-cardiac surgery. Sleep Med Rev 2001;5(2):129–37.
39. Cheatle MD, Savage SR. Informed consent in opioid therapy: a potential obligation and opportunity. J Pain Symptom Manage 2012;44(1):105–16.
40. Buysse DJ. Insomnia. JAMA 2013;309:706–16.
41. Roehrs T, Roth T. Insomnia pharmacotherapy. Neurotherapeutics 2012;9:728–38.
42. NIH State-of-the-science conference statement on manifestations and management of chronic insomnia in adults. NIH Consens State Sci Statements 2005; 22(2):1–30.
43. Bartusch SL, Sanders BJ, D'Alessio JG, et al. Clonazepam for the treatment of lancinating phantom limb pain. Clin J Pain 1996;12:59–62.
44. Menefee LA, Cohen MJ, Anderson WR, et al. Sleep disturbance and nonmalignant chronic pain: a comprehensive review of the literature. Pain Med 2000;1: 156–72.
45. King S, Strain J. Benzodiazepine use by chronic pain patients. Clin J Pain 1990; 6(2):143–7.
46. Glass J, Lanctôt KL, Herrmann N, et al. Sedative hypnotics in older people with insomnia: meta-analysis of risks and benefits. BMJ 2005;331:1169.
47. Roehrs T, Zorick FJ, Sicklesteel JM, et al. Effects of hypnotics on memory. J Clin Psychopharmacol 1983;3:310–3.
48. Licata SC, Rowlett JK. Abuse and dependence liability of benzodiazepine-type drugs: GABA(A) receptor modulation and beyond. Pharmacol Biochem Behav 2008;90(1):74–89.
49. Pollack M, Kinrys G, Krystal A, et al. Eszopiclone coadministered with escitalopram in patients with insomnia and comorbid generalized anxiety disorder. Arch Gen Psychiatry 2008;65:551–62.
50. Randall S, Roehrs TA, Roth T. Efficacy of eight months of nightly zolpidem: a prospective placebo-controlled study. Sleep 2012;35:1551–7.
51. Roth T, Walsh JK, Krystal A, et al. An evaluation of the efficacy and safety of eszopiclone over 12 months in patients with chronic primary insomnia. Sleep Med 2005;6:487–95.
52. Moldofsky H, Lue FA, Mously C, et al. The effect of zolpidem in patients with fibromyalgia: a dose ranging, double blind, placebo controlled, modified crossover study. J Rheumatol 1996;23:529–33.
53. Roth T, Price JM, Amato DA, et al. The effect of eszopiclone in patients with insomnia and coexisting rheumatoid arthritis: a pilot study. Prim Care Companion J Clin Psychiatry 2009;11:292–301.
54. Mason M, Cates CJ, Smith I. Effects of opioid, hypnotic and sedating medications on sleep-disordered breathing in adults with obstructive sleep apnoea. Cochrane Database Syst Rev 2015;(7):CD011090.

55. Darke S, Deady M, Duflou J. Toxicology and characteristics of deaths involving zolpidem in New South Wales, Australia 2001-2010. J Forensic Sci 2012;57(5): 1259–62.

56. Mayers AG, Baldwin DS. Antidepressants and their effect on sleep. Hum Psychopharmacol 2005;20:533–59.

57. Moulin DE, Clark AJ, Gilron I, et al. Pharmacological management of chronic neuropathic pain - consensus statement and guidelines from the Canadian Pain Society. Pain Res Manag 2007;12(1):13–21.

58. Shipley JE, Kupfer DJ, Griffin SJ, et al. Comparison of effects of desipramine and amitriptyline on EEG sleep of depressed patients. Psychopharmacology (Berl) 1985;85:14–22.

59. Sonntag A, Rothe B, Guldner J, et al. Trimipramine and imipramine exert different effects on the sleep EEG and on nocturnal hormone secretion during treatment of major depression. Depression 1996;4:1–13.

60. Gursky JT, Krahn LE. The effects of antidepressants on sleep: a review. Harv Rev Psychiatry 2000;8:298–306.

61. Boyle J, Eriksson ME, Gribble L, et al. Randomized, placebo-controlled comparison of amitriptyline, duloxetine, and pregabalin in patients with chronic diabetic peripheral neuropathic pain: impact on pain, polysomnographic sleep, daytime functioning, and quality of life. Diabetes Care 2012;35:2451–8.

62. Häuser W, Petzke F, Üçeyler N, et al. Comparative efficacy and acceptability of amitriptyline, duloxetine and milnacipran in fibromyalgia syndrome: a systematic review with meta-analysis. Rheumatology (Oxford) 2011;50:532–43.

63. McQuay HJ, Carroll D, Glynn CJ. Dose-response for analgesic effect of amitriptyline in chronic pain. Anaesthesia 1993;48:281–5.

64. McCall C, McCall WV. What is the role of sedating antidepressants, antipsychotics, and anticonvulsants in the management of insomnia? Curr Psychiatry Rep 2012;14(5):494–502.

65. Godfrey RG. A guide to the understanding and use of tricyclic antidepressants in the overall management of fibromyalgia and other chronic pain syndromes. Arch Intern Med 1996;156:1047–52.

66. Rosenbaum JF. Handbook of psychiatric drug therapy (Google eBook). Philadelphia: Lippincott Williams & Wilkins; 2009. p. 304.

67. Bossini L, Casolaro I, Koukouna D, et al. Off-label uses of trazodone: a review. Expert Opin Pharmacother 2012;13(12):1707–17.

68. Morillas-Arques P, Rodriguez-Lopez CM, Molina-Barea R, et al. Trazodone for the treatment of fibromyalgia: an open-label, 12-week study. BMC Musculoskelet Disord 2010;11:204.

69. Wilson RC. The use of low-dose trazodone in the treatment of painful diabetic neuropathy. J Am Podiatr Med Assoc 1999;89:468–71.

70. Walsh JK, Erman M, Erwin CW, et al. Subjective hypnotic efficacy of trazodone and zolpidem in DSMIII-R primary insomnia. Hum Psychopharmacol 1998;13: 191–8.

71. Kim S-W, Shin I-S, Kim J-M, et al. Effectiveness of mirtazapine for nausea and insomnia in cancer patients with depression. Psychiatry Clin Neurosci 2008;62: 75–83.

72. Bendtsen L, Jensen R. Mirtazapine is effective in the prophylactic treatment of chronic tension-type headache. Neurology 2004;62:1706–11.

73. Christodoulou C, Douzenis A, Moussas G, et al. Effectiveness of mirtazapine in the treatment of postherpetic neuralgia. J Pain Symptom Manage 2010;39:e3–6.

74. Nutt D, Law J. Treatment of cluster headache with mirtazapine. Headache 1999; 39:586–7.
75. Calandre EP, Rico-Villademoros F. The role of antipsychotics in the management of fibromyalgia. CNS Drugs 2012;26:135–53.
76. Krymchantowski AV, Jevoux C, Moreira PF. An open pilot study assessing the benefits of quetiapine for the prevention of migraine refractory to the combination of atenolol, nortriptyline, and flunarizine. Pain Med 2010;11:48–52.
77. Backonja M, Beydoun A, Edwards KR, et al. Gabapentin for the symptomatic treatment of painful neuropathy in patients with diabetes mellitus: a randomized controlled trial. JAMA 1998;280:1831–6.
78. Sabatowski R, Gálvez R, Cherry DA, et al. Pregabalin reduces pain and improves sleep and mood disturbances in patients with post-herpetic neuralgia: results of a randomised, placebo-controlled clinical trial. Pain 2004;109:26–35.
79. Mula M, Pini S, Cassano GB. The role of anticonvulsant drugs in anxiety disorders: a critical review of the evidence. J Clin Psychopharmacol 2007;27:263–72.
80. Sateia MJ, Kirby-Long P, Taylor JL. Efficacy and clinical safety of ramelteon: an evidence-based review. Sleep Med Rev 2008;12:319–32.
81. Wilhelmsen M, Amirian I, Reiter RJ, et al. Analgesic effects of melatonin: a review of current evidence from experimental and clinical studies. J Pineal Res 2011;51: 270–7.

Using Chronic Pain Outcomes Data to Improve Outcomes

Neel Mehta, MD[a], Charles E. Inturrisi, PhD[b], Susan D. Horn, PhD[c], Lisa R. Witkin, MD[a],*

KEYWORDS

- Practice-based evidence • Patient-reported outcomes • Outcomes data collection
- Analysis of patient data • Quality improvement • Mobile health
- Electronic health record integration

KEY POINTS

- A major impediment to the advancement in research and clinical care in pain management is the difficulty and limited acceptance of objectively measuring and tracking pain treatment outcomes.
- Outcome assessments should be validated, standardized, and implemented with minimal burden on both the patient and health care team.
- In the near future, integrating patient-reported outcome (PRO) data into electronic health records (EHRs) and collecting and sharing mobile health (mHealth) data will produce new models of health care delivery, with the potential to improve outcomes assessments as well as quality and cost-effectiveness of chronic pain treatments.

INTRODUCTION

Chronic pain is one of the most common and most serious conditions affecting the health, quality of life, and productivity of Americans. It exerts a substantial social and economic burden on both the affected individual and society as a whole. According to an Institute of Medicine (IOM) report in 2011, more than 100 million Americans suffer with chronic pain, costing the nation more than $600 billion.[1] One of the most commonly studied categories of chronic pain involves low back pain, which affects

Disclosures: The Tri-Institutional Pain Registry was developed with the support of grant RC2 DA028928 from NIDA and is currently supported in part by a grant from Purdue Pharm, Ltd. No authors have any other conflicts of interest/disclosures to report.
[a] Department of Anesthesiology, Weill Cornell Pain Medicine, Weill Cornell Medical College, 1305 York Avenue, 10th Floor, New York, NY 10021, USA; [b] Department of Pharmacology, Weill Cornell Medical College, 1300 York Avenue, LC-519A, New York, NY 10065, USA; [c] Department of Population Health Sciences, Health System Innovation and Research Division, University of Utah, School of Medicine, 295 Chipeta Way, Room 1N461, Salt Lake City, UT 84108, USA
* Corresponding author.
E-mail address: Lrw9003@med.cornell.edu

Anesthesiology Clin 34 (2016) 395–408
http://dx.doi.org/10.1016/j.anclin.2016.01.009
1932-2275/16/$ – see front matter © 2016 Elsevier Inc. All rights reserved.

more than 31 million Americans annually[2] and can lead to nearly 149 million missed work days per year.[3] Treatment costs for this condition surpass $100 billion annually and have increased nearly 75% since 1987.[3]

Increases in these costs are multifactorial: an aging population with longer life spans leads to greater utilization of care, a decreased willingness to live with pain (due to patient preference and marketing campaigns of health care providers and institutions), and an increase in patient expectations. As a result, increased utilization is manifested in increased costly drug utilization, increased imaging and diagnostic tests, and ultimately increased injections and surgical procedures. Despite the best of intentions by providers, this increase in utilization and associated costs has not necessarily improved outcomes.[3]

Moreover, chronic pain treatments are highly variable between different pain management centers and even different practitioners within the same pain practice. A major impediment to the advancement of research and clinical care in pain management is the difficulty and limited acceptance of objectively measuring and tracking pain treatment outcomes.

Despite the scientific advances in understanding of pain physiology, anatomy, and biochemistry, along with the development of novel analgesic medications and interventions, chronic pain often remains poorly controlled. Large gaps exist in the knowledge base of the effectiveness of drug and nondrug interventions for chronic pain management, particularly due to the lack of longer-term outcomes data of the most commonly used interventions for chronic pain management.[4,5]

The IOM report in 2011 recommended a paradigm shift in the way pain is assessed and managed at the patient-provider level as well as how information is gathered and disseminated to fill the large gaps in the knowledge base.[1] The IOM report emphasized a need for greater development and use of patient outcome registries that can support point-of-care treatment decision making as well as for aggregation of large numbers of patients to enable assessment of the safety and effectiveness of therapies.[1]

HEALTH CARE ECONOMICS

The proper goal for any health care delivery system is to improve the value of care delivered to patients. Value in health care is measured in terms of the patient outcomes achieved per dollar expended. More care and more expensive care are not necessarily better care. To properly manage value, both outcomes and cost must be measured at the patient level. Measured outcomes and cost must encompass the entire cycle of care for a patient's particular medical condition, which often involves a team with multiple specialties performing multiple interventions from diagnosis to treatment to ongoing management. The magnitude of the opportunity to reduce costs and deliver improved outcomes—without limiting access to necessary care—is astounding.

The inability to properly measure cost and compare cost with outcomes is at the root of the incentive problem in health care and has severely retarded the shift to more effective reimbursement approaches. Poor measurement of cost and outcomes also means that effective and efficient providers go unrewarded, whereas inefficient ones have little incentive to improve. Institutions may be penalized when the improvements they make in treatments and processes reduce the need for highly reimbursed services.[6]

In pain management, the difficulty lies in the chronic nature of patients' suffering. There is ample evidence of multimodal treatment providing greater long-term efficacy in care and concern over overutilization in interventional and opioid treatments. The presence of large-scale randomized controlled trials (RCTs) has been limited at best, however, often questioning efficacies of established treatment options. Despite the growing influence of lists of empirically supported therapies, there are concerns about the design and conduct of this body of research, including limitations inherent in the requirements of RCTs that favor those pain treatments that define problems and outcome in terms of uncomplicated symptoms, similar to the struggle with studying psychotherapy treatments. These may be due to criteria for patient selection, lack of integration with research on long-term pain care process and effectiveness studies, limited outcome criteria, ethical dilemmas in placebo treatment in painful conditions, and lack of controls for experimenter bias.

It is agreed that RCTs have an important place in outcomes research but can also place restrictions on what and how pain therapy can be studied. There is a need for large-scale pain treatment outcomes research based on designs that allow for inclusion of process variables and the study of the effects of those idiographic approaches to therapy that do not lend themselves to RCT designs, especially in pain treatments where outcomes are not defined or understood solely in terms of symptom reduction.[7]

UTILIZING DATA TO IMPROVE EFFICIENCY AND QUALITY

US health care systems continue to expand the use of big data creatively and effectively to drive efficiency and quality in the sector that creates more than $300 billion in value every year. Intermountain Healthcare in Utah, a health care system that is self-insured, is often cited for health care excellence in the development of clinical integration. Their health care delivery research team created a system involving both medical providers and administrators to gather and analyze data to develop protocols, integrating the data with evidence from the literature to create evidence-based medicine guidelines applicable at the local level. The stated goal was to "Make it easy to do it right," allowing decision support to help guide best care, in a more efficient manner.

In 1996, after adopting these programs as part of clinical integration, they began to implement the processes and concurrently developed an outcome tracking system that held personnel accountable. They developed champions who integrated recommendations from the literature, analyzed local data results, and made suggestions for constant improvement from the end users, deemed *neat ideas*. Although the protocols were not mandatory, those users who repeatedly deviated from the plan were asked to provide support for their decisions, and the feedback was used to further improve protocols. Information technology support was crucial in development of physician education, user friendliness, and real-time data.

Together these changes brought about not only cost savings but also overall improved patient outcomes. Increased savings for the payers and shared reward for providers in Intermountain Healthcare's vertically integrated system was achieved; however, the important message is that the system is fluid, with constant surveillance to tighten and improve existing protocols or create new ones. This is a model that can and should be emulated and replicated.

BEGINNINGS OF TRACKING PAIN OUTCOMES ON A NATIONAL LEVEL

The 2011 IOM report summarized findings and recommendations on how to address the gaps in pain prevention, care, education, and research. The report identified the following recommendations related to service delivery and reimbursement in the areas of pain management[1]:

- Develop strategies for reducing barriers to pain care.
- Promote and enable self-management of pain.
- Support collaboration between pain specialists and primary care clinicians, including referral to pain centers when appropriate.

- Improve the collection and reporting of data on pain.
- Expand patient and public education, including prevention.
- Revise reimbursement policies to foster coordinated and evidence-based pain care.

With greater collection of data, learning, and outcome measures, evidence can guide health care providers to individualize their pain care most appropriately. These conclusions were presented to government bodies with the anticipation of making meaningful inclusions into future government programs and regulations a national priority, highlighting the burden of pain in human lives both financially and socially.

THE AFFORDABLE CARE ACT

The Affordable Care Act (ACA) was developed at a time of rapidly escalating concern regarding health care costs and quality of care. As annual health care spending approached 20% of GDP, with double-digit inflationary rates, these costs of care were deemed unsustainable. Chronic pain is a major driver for visits to physicians, a common reason for taking medications, a significant cause of disability, and a key factor in quality of life and productivity. Given the IOM's recommendations related to improved service delivery, ACA provisions that focus on improved coordination, alignment of incentives, and quality may also have an impact on pain care. These include provisions, such as Accountable Care Organizations, Value-Based Purchasing, and the Multi-payer Advanced Primary Care Practice Demonstration.[8]

The ACA contains 3 key provisions to increase understanding and improve the delivery of evidence-based care for pain management (**Table 1**).[9]

In response to the recommendations of the IOM report, the Interagency Pain Research Coordinating Committee (IPRCC) developed a draft report of a National Pain Strategy (http://iprcc.nih.gov/National_Pain_Strategy/NPS_Main.htm). As the draft indicates, "Guided and coordinated by an oversight panel, expert working groups explored six important areas of need identified in the IOM recommendations—population research, prevention and care, disparities, service delivery and reimbursement, professional education and training, and public awareness and communication. The working groups comprised people from a broad array of relevant public and private organizations, including health care providers, insurers, and people with pain and their advocates." The draft report summaries the National Pain Strategy as follows: "If the objectives of the National Pain Strategy are achieved, the nation would see a decrease in prevalence across the continuum of pain, from acute, to chronic, to high-impact chronic pain, and across the life span from pediatric through geriatric populations, to end of life, which would reduce the burden of pain for individuals, families, and society as a whole. Americans experiencing pain—across this broad continuum—would have timely access to a care system that meets their biopsychosocial needs and takes into account individual preferences, risks, and social contexts. In other words, they would receive patient-centered care." Public comment on the draft ended May 20, 2015 and the final report is being completed.

Thus far, the Centers for Medicare & Medicaid Services (CMS) has moved toward tracking of pain (**Table 2**).[8]

Furthermore, CMS is also engaged in demonstration projects and policy changes that could impact reimbursement and delivery of pain care.

Bundled Payment for Care Improvement Initiative

CMS is conducting several care and reimbursement demonstrations to encourage coordination among providers and more efficient use of services. CMS began the

Table 1		
Affordable Care Act provisions		
	Provision	**Goal**
Section 4305	Requires the US HHS to partner with the IOM to convene the Conference on Pain	• Evaluating the adequacy of pain-related care and treatments in the general population and among identified groups • Identifying barriers to pain care • Establishing an agenda for both the public and private sectors that reduces barriers and improves pain research, education, and care
Section 409J	Establishes the IPRCC to coordinate all pain-related research within HHS and other federal agencies	• Developing a summary of advances in pain care research relevant to the diagnosis, prevention, and treatment of pain and diseases and disorders associated with pain • Identifying research gaps in the symptoms and causes of pain • Providing suggestions on how best to disseminate information on pain care
Section 759	Encourages HHS to award grants, cooperative agreements, and contracts to health profession schools, hospices, and other public and private entities	Development and implementation of programs that provide pain care education and training to health care professionals

Abbreviation: HHS, Department of Health and Human Services.

Adapted from Lausch K. Pain related care and the Affordable Care Act: summary of common practices. 2014. Available at: http://www.chrt.org/publication/pain-related-care-and-the-affordable-care-act-summary-of-common-practices/-accordion-section-5.

Bundled Payments for Care Improvement initiative in 2013. The 3-year initiative uses 4 broadly defined models to test the use of bundle payments (paid either prospectively or retrospectively) for 48 episodes of care, such as spinal fusions. The 4 models of care span acute and postacute providers and services.[10]

Chronic Care Management Services

CMS continues to examine how care management is reimbursed. In 2015, Medicare intends to start providing a separate reimbursement for non–face-to-face chronic care management services for beneficiaries with multiple (2 or more) significant chronic conditions. Currently, this payment is bundled into payments for evaluation and management services, but many physicians believe it does not adequately describe the services provided. CMS hopes the policy improves the management and decreases the costs of chronic diseases. The separate reimbursement for non–face-to-face chronic care management services is expected to be further defined via the Physician Fee Schedule rulemaking process for calendar year 2015.[11]

CENTERS FOR MEDICARE & MEDICAID SERVICES OUTCOMES AND OPIOID PRESCRIPTION PROGRAMS

CMS has been taking actions in the chronic pain space for some time now, most recently in the area of chronic opioid usage. With evidence pointing to increased diversion associated with increased prescription opioid availability and greater abuse and

Table 2
Examples of Centers for Medicare & Medicaid Services quality measures

Examples of Centers for Medicare & Medicaid Services Quality Measures	Measure	Description
Home Health Compare	Improvement in pain interfering with activity	Percentage of home health episodes of care during which a patient's frequency of pain when moving around improved
Home Health Quality Reporting	Pain assessment conducted	Percentage of home health episodes of care in which the patient was assessed for pain, using a standardized pain assessment tool, at start/resumption of care
Hospital Compare	Pain management (summary measure)	Patients who reported that their pain was "Always" well controlled
Medicare and Medicaid EHR Incentive Program for Eligible Professionals	166v2: use of imaging studies for low back pain	Percentage of patients 18–50 y of age with a diagnosis of low back pain who did not have an imaging study (plain radiograph, MRI, CT scan) within 28 d of diagnosis
Medicare Part C Plan Finder/Star Rating	C13—care for older adults – pain screening	Percent of plan members who had a pain screening or pain management plan at least once during the year (this information about pain screening or pain management is collected for Medicare Special Needs Plans only. Some Special Needs Plans are for people with certain chronic diseases and conditions, some are for people who have both Medicare and Medicaid, and some are for people who live in an institution such as a nursing home.)
Medicare Physician Quality Reporting System	Measure #131 (NQF 0420): pain assessment and follow-up	Percentage of visits for patients aged 18 y and older with documentation of a pain assessment through discussion with the patient, including the use of a standardized tool(s) on each visit AND documentation of a follow-up plan when pain is present
Physician Value-Based Payment Modifier	Measure #131 (NQF 0420): pain assessment and follow-up	Percentage of visits for patients aged 18 y and older with documentation of a pain assessment through discussion with the patient including the use of a standardized tool(s) on each visit AND documentation of a follow-up plan when pain is present
Physician Value-Based Payment Modifier	Lower back pain: repeat imaging studies	Percentage of patients with back pain who received inappropriate imaging studies in the absence of red flags or progressive symptoms (overuse measure, lower performance is better)

Data from Lausch, K. Pain-Related Care and the Affordable Care Act: Summary of Common Practices. Ann Arbor (MI): The Center for Healthcare Research & Transformation (CHRT); 2014.

adverse event rates with long-term opioid usage, outcomes measures have led to tighter policies for opioid prescriptions through both public and private payers. They are concerned about the associated costs and risks for abuse and addiction, evident in policies commonly used by payers, including quantity limits, prior authorizations, step therapy, and lock-in programs (members are restricted to a single pharmacy and/or prescriber group). In Michigan, for example, Blue Cross Blue Shield requires documentation that members have experienced treatment failure of or intolerance to 2 other long-acting opioids before they can be prescribed extended-release oxycodone.

PATIENT-REPORTED OUTCOME MEASURES

There are many PROs that can be used to provide information about severity of pain and its impact on patients' physical and psychological wellbeing. Outcome assessment tools can be generic measures of health or disease specific, such as for chronic pain. The Initiative on Methods, Measurement, and Pain Assessment in Clinical Trials (IMMPACT) group recommends several key domains that should be considered in selecting outcome measures for clinical trials, including pain, physical functioning, emotional functioning, participant ratings of global improvement, symptoms and adverse events, disposition, and reasons for premature withdrawal from a trial.[12]

The Patient Reported Outcome Measurement Information System (PROMIS) is a dynamic tool developed through National Institutes of Health funding that is psychometrically validated and efficiently assesses PROs across a wide range of chronic diseases and demographic characteristics.[13,14] PROMIS can improve PRO measurement quality and precision, in part through utilizing item response theory (IRT). IRT is a method commonly used in educational testing that creates statistical models based on IRT-produced scores (calibrations) associated with answers to questions. These calibrations provide computer software with information to select the most informative follow-up question. This computer software is called computer adaptive testing (CAT) because the content of the assessment, or questions asked, adapts to a patient based on responses to the previous question.

The PROMIS measures outcomes across physical, social, mental, and global health domains. To enhance generalizability and interpretability, all PROMIS measures have been centered on a sample that is representative of the US general population in important demographics (ie, race/ethnicity, age, and gender).[14,15] To maintain continuity with previous research, crosswalk approaches have been developed that can be used to transform Brief Pain Inventory (BPI) pain interference scores to PROMIS pain interference short form scores.[15]

TRI-INSTITUTIONAL PAIN REGISTRY

The Tri-Institutional Pain Registry (TPR) is a longitudinal chronic pain patient registry that includes patients from pain medicine clinics of Weill Cornell Medical College (WCMC), Memorial Sloan Kettering Cancer Center (MSKCC), and Hospital for Special Surgery (HSS), all located in New York City. The goals of the TPR are to identify patient characteristics and treatments that are associated with better or worse outcomes for TPR patients. In addition, the TPR shares information that results from analysis of TPR data with clinicians who are part of the TPR, with the pain community in the form of publications and guidelines, and with supporters (public and private) of this project. The primary goal of the TPR is as part of a quality improvement program utilizing both the point-of care data as well as the aggregate analysis of the data.

The TPR was developed using a model of comparative effectiveness research called practice-based evidence (PBE).[16] PBE is an observational method for determining which patient characteristics and treatments are associated with better or worse outcomes in real-world patients. PBE measures effectiveness, that is, For which patients does it work? The TPR is not measuring efficacy, that is, Does it work? TPR data elements are, wherever possible, part of routine EHR documentation and include (1) process factors (treatments) for example, medications—current and past—and all procedures, and (2) patient factors, diagnostic codes, demographics, and medical, surgical, and social histories. The decision on which data elements to collect and analyze directly involves point-of-care clinicians who meet regularly with TPR staff where these decisions are made. This bottom-up rather than a top-down approach fosters clinician commitment. The TPR also sought guidance from expert pain researchers that comprise its scientific advisory board and conducted pilot testing of elements and sought feedback from clinic staff. It was essential to work with clinicians to standardize codes (International Classification of Diseases, Ninth Revision [now International Classification of Diseases, Tenth Revision] and Current Procedural Terminology) that are used across the sites (eg, approximately 339 pain-related codes are used by the clinicians) and to standardize medication capture and conversion of opioids to morphine equivalents.

PROs are also essential data elements and are standardized across the 3 sites. The TPR agreed to use validated outcome documentation tools. When the development of the TPR began in 2009, the BPI[17] was already in use at the MSKCC site and the Condensed Memorial Symptom Assessment Schedule (CMSAS)[18] had been developed at MSKCC. Therefore, it was agreed that at each of the 3 sites, the BPI that includes measures of pain, subjective effects, and pain-related functional changes[17] and the CMSAS that measures treatment-related adverse effects[18] would be used. In addition, it was agreed to use the EQ-5D, a measure of general health status,[19] and the Current Opioid Misuse Measure,[20] which measures aberrant opioid-related behaviors.

Data generated by these surveys are stored in WebCore (MSKCC), a secure central data storage computer, and are available in real time to the clinicians in the clinic and, subsequently, in a Health Insurance Portability and Accountability Act (HIPAA) compliant format in Excel or other formats to the collaborators at the University of Utah (discussed later).

To minimize sample biases, participation in the TPR is standard operating procedure (standard of care) so that every patient who attends the clinic twice, with visits separated by at least 3 months, is denoted a "chronic pain patient" and is entered into the TPR and asked to complete a survey at each encounter. It is essential to confirm with the local institutional review board that these activities are part of a quality improvement program so that these activities can be conducted with a waiver of informed consent and of HIPAA consent. In addition, the institutional review board needs to be informed about data sharing with secondary sites, including sponsors, and the development and dissemination of guidelines and publications.

Data Collection and Storage

Fig. 1 shows interactions among the components of the TPR using the WCMC site to represent the activities at each site. The clinical data administrator (CDA) coordinates activities necessary among the patient, the clinician, WebCore, and Epic (EHR) that constitute the data sources for the TPR. The CDA enters a patient in WebCore and confirms that the patient is also in Epic (see Fig. 1). The patient completes the outcomes survey at the clinic visit using an iPad or within 48 hours prior to the clinic visit via an e-mail link. The iPad is linked to WebCore and as soon as the survey is

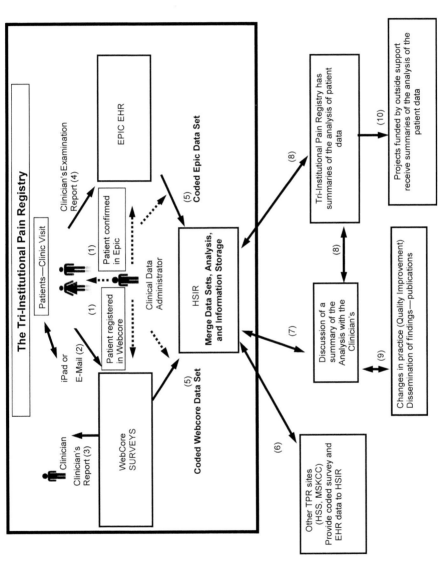

Fig. 1. A diagram of the workflow, including the collection, merging, storage, analysis, and dissemination of registry data by the Tri-Institutional Pain Registry.

completed by the patient, a summary of patient responses for the current visit and the previous visit is available to the clinician as a printout, called the clinician's report. The clinician can use survey information to initiate a conversation with the patient and to develop a treatment plan. This engages both clinician and patient in participation with the survey. Subsequently, the clinician's report is scanned into Epic by the CDA and becomes part of each patient's EHR. The patient encounter also results in a clinician's examination report (eg, diagnoses, medications, and other clinic visit information) that is entered into Epic. Clinicians can review all WebCore surveys for their patients and can follow the outcomes of treatments for individual patients.

Merging Patient Data from Different Electronic Systems

Collaborators at the Health System Innovation and Research (HSIR) program of University of Utah School of Medicine, Salt Lake City, Utah, host the database and merge PRO data captured in WebCore with clinical data captured in Epic to form a complete coded data set for the TPR database (see **Fig. 1**). Merged data from WebCore and Epic have a common coded patient identification that links them. Coded data are transferred to HSIR using the WCMC secure file transfer system and merged by HSIR and added to the TPR database. HSIR maintains both a separate WCMC merged coded database and, when requested, merges databases or elements of databases from MSKCC and HSS with the WCMC database.

Data Analysis and Dissemination

Descriptive statistics are used to describe outcomes, status of patients, and treatments at initial visit and each follow-up visit. Longitudinal regression analyses are used to determine treatments associated with outcomes, controlling for patient differences.[16] The analysis process is an iterative one where certain analyses are conducted and summary data are shared with the clinicians (see **Fig. 1**). Suggestions are made for other analyses that might identify (or reject) additional important associations and predictors. The TPR together with HSIR decide the additional analyses that will be conducted by HSIR and this process continues until agreement is reached that the major associations and predictors have been identified that define the objectives of the analysis. Summary data are then disseminated to clinicians to be used for quality improvement and, together with clinicians, manuscripts are prepared for publication. For projects funded by outside support, selected deidentified summaries of the data analysis are made available to the sponsors.

INTEGRATION INTO ELECTRONIC HEALTH RECORDS

A future area of improvement in chronic pain outcomes data collection is real-time integration of PRO into the EHR. EHR integration offers many potential advantages. EHR integration allows the coordination of PRO administration with meaningful clinic events, such as scheduled medical visits, to maximize clinical utility.[13] Optimally designed EHR-integrated systems can provide real-time delivery of PRO results for clinician decision support and can enhance effective management by alerting clinicians to significant symptoms (ie, severely abnormal results or patient concerns). EHR integration can also be designed to provide automated triage to specialty providers, when appropriate, for example, to social work providers for psychosocial concerns, to health educators for information, and to dietitians for nutrition-related concerns.[13] This enhances coordination of care and can support multidisciplinary sites in integrating their specialties in a meaningful way, all with the goal of improving the comprehensive management of chronic pain patients. The clinical integration of

PROMIS CAT administration, scoring, and reporting within an EHR system has been used successfully.[13]

INTEGRATING MOBILE TECHNOLOGY

More than 125 million people in the United States own smartphones, and smartphones account for more than 50% of mobile phone sales in the United States.[21] The widespread use of mobile technology and its flexibility, simplicity, and increasing affordability make it impossible to ignore as a novel approach to significantly improve pain management. Smartphones are increasingly used in research and may offer an opportunity to develop interventions at a lower cost and with decreased provider burden to help patients monitor and manage their pain symptoms.[22]

Smartphones have been used to improve pain and health outcomes through the use of specialized software applications (apps) for assessing pain symptoms, facilitating communication between patients and providers, tracking outcomes (physical functioning and activity levels), delivering information, and tracking behaviors. mHealth approaches can use a combination of active and passive functions to collect both objective and subjective outcomes data.[23] These data can be collected outside the clinical setting, allowing for more effective monitoring and more accurate reporting between office visits, effectively bridging the current gaps in chronic disease management.

In terms of chronic pain, apps have been developed that allow patients to record diary entries between office visits and allow therapists to send tailored text messages to patients.[24–27] In nonpain settings, smartphones have been used in RCTs to track physical activity,[28] monitor weight loss,[22] and improve nutrition and encourage weight loss.[29] Studies examining mHealth strategies to manage chronic medical illnesses and psychiatric disorders have found that mHealth delivery is feasible, acceptable, and efficacious.[30–33]

mHealth may also allow for innovative treatment delivery mechanisms, such as promoting patient behavior change through real-time feedback, or providing medical advice, automatically, based on patterns in PRO data, which can improve self-management.[24] These applications of mHealth have been shown to decrease preventable health care utilization in certain chronic pain populations, including a study of patients with sickle cell disease who require adequate and early pain treatment.[24] Moreover, mHealth can decrease barriers to care (eg, provide instruction in cognitive-behavioral therapy methods that improve access to behavioral pain therapies).[23] Additional health care benefits include improved communication among professionals and between patients and professionals due to enriched additional data—possibly leading to reduced costs and improved patient care.[34] In the near future, collecting and sharing mHealth data between patients and multiple authorized stakeholders will likely produce new models of health care delivery and improved treatments for chronic pain care.[23]

Despite the widespread availability of mobile technology, current apps are limited by the scarce participation of health care providers in their creation and minimal data on their efficacy.[35] Dr L. Wallace and Dhingra conducted a systematic review of 222 unique pain-related mobile apps and found that most provided the patient with pain diaries, exercises, and pain-coping strategies to help manage stress, moderate emotional reactions, and maintain a balanced lifestyle.[36] Approximately two-thirds of these apps, however, were not designed or edited by licensed health care providers; only 27% of the apps had confirmed participation by a physician and 8% by a nonphysician health care provider.[37] Although these apps may have significant potential, the development by non–health care professionals may limit their validity and effectiveness.

There is a lack of guidance on how to develop apps that are evidence based and most suitable for particular users. Rosser and colleagues[38] described several core characteristics that a panel of clinicians and chronic pain patients believed are important to incorporate into the design of a pain management app. Important characteristics include supporting awareness of behavioral patterns, encouraging personal goals, and providing access to a real-time therapist.

Despite the numerous potential advantages, there are some disadvantages to consider. mHealth technology may not be user centered, and the resulting amount of data could overwhelm providers and fragment care delivery because it is currently poorly integrated with EHRs. Moreover, more research is needed in terms of the effects of making patients' mHealth data available to family, health care providers, and/or other approved stakeholders. Lastly, compliance is a significant barrier, because it may decrease over time. Efforts to improve long-term compliance with apps may include automated systems to deliver cues to patients, directly following up with patients who have not entered data, integrating positive reinforcements for use (eg, badges and increased feedback from providers), instilling entertainment value (gamification), and incorporating a social network into the app.[39]

SUMMARY

The ultimate goal of registry data collection is to develop an evidenced-based system that efficiently and effectively improves chronic pain treatment quality and cost-effectiveness.[40] This effort should be coordinated—ideally across the nation and across primary and multidisciplinary specialties managing chronic pain—with regard to the selection of outcome measurements, how data sets are organized, and sharing of data for research purposes.[40] The meaningful use of PRO requires a system that provides validated, precise, accurate, and robust symptom assessment that is brief, minimizing burden on both patients and health care teams, and maximizes feasibility for quality improvement and research. Moreover, the system needs to allow for iterative modifications, as necessary, and ongoing data analysis to help direct individual patient care as well as for population health efforts.

REFERENCES

1. Institute of Medicine (US) Committee on Advancing Pain Research, Care, and Education. Relieving Pain in America: A Blueprint for Transforming Prevention, Care, Education, and Research. Washington, DC: National Academies Press (US); 2011. Available from: http://www.ncbi.nlm.nih.gov/books/NBK91497/.

2. Shaw WS, Linton SJ, Pransky G. Reducing sickness absence from work due to low back pain: how well do intervention strategies match modifiable risk factors? J Occup Rehabil 2006;16(4):591–605.

3. Martin BI, Deyo RA, Mirza SK, et al. Expenditures and health status among adults with back and neck problems. JAMA 2008;299(6):656–64.

4. Reid MC, Bennett DA, Chen WG, et al. Improving the pharmacologic management of pain in older adults: identifying the research gaps and methods to address them. Pain Med 2011;12(9):1336–57.

5. Bruehl S, Apkarian AV, Ballantyne JC, et al. Personalized medicine and opioid analgesic prescribing for chronic pain: opportunities and challenges. J Pain 2013;14(2):103–13.

6. Kaplan RS, Porter ME. How to solve the cost crisis in health care. Harv Bus Rev 2011;89(9):46–52, 54, 56-61 passim.
7. Shean G. Limitations of randomized control designs in psychotherapy research. Advances in Psychiatry 2014;2014:5.
8. Lausch K. Pain-Related Care and the Affordable Care Act: Summary of Common Practices. The Center for Healthcare Research & Transformation (CHRT). 2014. Available at: http://www.chrt.org/publication/pain-related-care-and-the-affordable-care-act-summary-of-common-practices/-accordion-section-5.
9. Manchikanti L, Caraway D, Parr AT, et al. Patient Protection and Affordable Care Act of 2010: reforming the health care reform for the new decade. Pain Physician 2011;14(1):E35–67.
10. Doran JP, Zabinski SJ. Bundled payment initiatives for Medicare and non-Medicare total joint arthroplasty patients at a community hospital: bundles in the real world. J Arthroplasty 2015;30(3):353–5.
11. Thompson CA. CMS explains Medicare payment for chronic care management services. Am J Health Syst Pharm 2015;72(7):514–5.
12. Turk DC, Dworkin RH, Allen RR, et al. Core outcome domains for chronic pain clinical trials: IMMPACT recommendations. Pain 2003;106(3):337–45.
13. Wagner LI, Schink J, Bass M, et al. Bringing PROMIS to practice: brief and precise symptom screening in ambulatory cancer care. Cancer 2015;121(6):927–34.
14. Amtmann D, Cook KF, Jensen MP, et al. Development of a PROMIS item bank to measure pain interference. Pain 2010;150(1):173–82.
15. Askew RL, Kim J, Chung H, et al. Development of a crosswalk for pain interference measured by the BPI and PROMIS pain interference short form. Qual Life Res 2013;22(10):2769–76.
16. Horn SD, DeJong G, Deutscher D. Practice-based evidence research in rehabilitation: an alternative to randomized controlled trials and traditional observational studies. Arch Phys Med Rehabil 2012;93(8 Suppl):S127–37.
17. Mendoza T, Mayne T, Rublee D, et al. Reliability and validity of a modified brief pain inventory short form in patients with osteoarthritis. Eur J Pain 2006;10(4):353–61.
18. Chang VT, Hwang SS, Kasimis B, et al. Shorter symptom assessment instruments: the Condensed Memorial Symptom Assessment Scale (CMSAS). Cancer Invest 2004;22(4):526–36.
19. Hurst NP, Kind P, Ruta D, et al. Measuring health-related quality of life in rheumatoid arthritis: validity, responsiveness and reliability of EuroQol (EQ-5D). Br J Rheumatol 1997;36(5):551–9.
20. Butler SF, Budman SH, Fernandez KC, et al. Development and validation of the current opioid misuse measure. Pain 2007;130(1–2):144–56.
21. Barr C, Marois M, Sim I, et al. The PREEMPT study - evaluating smartphone-assisted n-of-1 trials in patients with chronic pain: study protocol for a randomized controlled trial. Trials 2015;16:67.
22. Pellegrini CA, Duncan JM, Moller AC, et al. A smartphone-supported weight loss program: design of the ENGAGED randomized controlled trial. BMC Public Health 2012;12:1041.
23. Richardson JE, Reid MC. The promises and pitfalls of leveraging mobile health technology for pain care. Pain Med 2013;14(11):1621–6.
24. Schnall R, Okoniewski A, Tiase V, et al. Using text messaging to assess adolescents' health information needs: an ecological momentary assessment. J Med Internet Res 2013;15(3):e54.

25. Stinson JN, Petroz GC, Tait G, et al. e-Ouch: usability testing of an electronic chronic pain diary for adolescents with arthritis. Clin J Pain 2006;22(3): 295–305.

26. Stinson JN, Stevens BJ, Feldman BM, et al. Construct validity of a multidimensional electronic pain diary for adolescents with arthritis. Pain 2008;136(3): 281–92.

27. Kristjansdottir OB, Fors EA, Eide E, et al. A smartphone-based intervention with diaries and therapist feedback to reduce catastrophizing and increase functioning in women with chronic widespread pain. Part 2: 11-month follow-up results of a randomized trial. J Med Internet Res 2013;15(3):e72.

28. Glynn LG, Hayes PS, Casey M, et al. SMART MOVE - a smartphone-based intervention to promote physical activity in primary care: study protocol for a randomized controlled trial. Trials 2013;14:157.

29. Duncan MJ, Vandelanotte C, Rosenkranz RR, et al. Effectiveness of a website and mobile phone based physical activity and nutrition intervention for middle-aged males: trial protocol and baseline findings of the ManUp Study. BMC Public Health 2012;12:656.

30. Somers TJ, Abernethy AP, Edmond SN, et al. A pilot study of a mobile health pain coping skills training protocol for patients with persistent cancer pain. J Pain Symptom Manage 2015;50(4):553–8.

31. Abernethy AP, Zafar SY, Uronis H, et al. Validation of the patient care monitor (Version 2.0): a review of system assessment instrument for cancer patients. J Pain Symptom Manage 2010;40(4):545–58.

32. Fortner B, Okon T, Schwartzberg L, et al. The cancer care monitor: psychometric content evaluation and pilot testing of a computer administered system for symptom screening and quality of life in adult cancer patients. J Pain Symptom Manage 2003;26(6):1077–92.

33. Lorig K, Holman H. Arthritis self-efficacy scales measure self-efficacy. Arthritis Care Res 1998;11(3):155–7.

34. Reynoldson C, Stones C, Allsop M, et al. Assessing the quality and usability of smartphone apps for pain self-management. Pain Med 2014;15(6): 898–909.

35. Christiansen S, Gupta A. Can mobile technology improve treatment of chronic pain? Pain Med 2014;15(8):1434–5.

36. Wallace LS, Dhingra LK. A systematic review of smartphone applications for chronic pain available for download in the United States. J Opioid Manag 2014;10(1):63–8.

37. Rosser BA, Eccleston C. Smartphone applications for pain management. J Telemed Telecare 2011;17(6):308–12.

38. Rosser BA, McCullagh P, Davies R, et al. Technology-mediated therapy for chronic pain management: the challenges of adapting behavior change interventions for delivery with pervasive communication technology. Telemed J E Health 2011;17(3):211–6.

39. Jonassaint CR, Shah N, Jonassaint J, et al. Usability and feasibility of an mHealth intervention for monitoring and managing pain symptoms in sickle cell disease: the sickle cell disease mobile application to record symptoms via technology (SMART). Hemoglobin 2015;39(3):162–8.

40. Witkin LR, Farrar JT, Ashburn MA. Can assessing chronic pain outcomes data improve outcomes? Pain Med 2013;14(6):779–91.

State Policies Regulating the Practice of Pain Management

Statutes, Rules, and Guidelines
That Shape Pain Care

Robert K. Twillman, PhD[a],*, Aaron M. Gilson, MS, MSSW, PhD[b],
Kathryn N. Duensing, JD[a],1

KEYWORDS

- Pain policy • Dosage thresholds • Clinical practice guidelines
- Rules and regulations • Pain management

KEY POINTS

- Statutes, rules/regulations, and guidelines guiding pain management practice are found in nearly every state and profoundly affect pain care.
- Although there is some uniformity across these policies, unique features can be found in nearly all categories of included provisions.
- These policies are intended to help minimize opioid misuse, abuse, addiction, diversion, and related overdoses but have not yet been proved to work.
- Future efforts to develop pain management policy should seek to maximize intended consequences while minimizing negative unintended consequences for people with pain.

INTRODUCTION

Over the past 2 decades, pain management in the United States has increasingly come to rely on opioid analgesics as a primary treatment. As a result, there has been a sharp increase in opioid prescribing, with opioid analgesic prescriptions, by weight, quadrupling since 1999.[1] Concomitantly, there has been a dramatic increase in overdose deaths involving prescription opioids, with those rates also nearly

Disclosure Statement: Dr R.K. Twillman is a consultant and speaker for Indivior. Dr A.M. Gilson and Ms K.N. Duensing have nothing to disclose.
[a] American Academy of Pain Management, 975 Morning Star Drive, Suite A, Sonora, CA 95370, USA; [b] Pain & Policy Studies Group, Carbone Cancer Center, University of Wisconsin, 1300 University Avenue, MSC 6152, Madison, WI 53706, USA
[1] Present Address: 57 Auburn Avenue Southeast, Grand Rapids, MI 49506.
* Corresponding author. 975 Morning Star Drive, Suite A, Sonora, CA 95370.
E-mail address: btwillman@aapainmanage.org

Anesthesiology Clin 34 (2016) 409–424
http://dx.doi.org/10.1016/j.anclin.2016.01.010   anesthesiology.theclinics.com

quadrupling between 1999 and 2008.[2] Although virtually nothing more is known about the circumstances of these overdoses, numerous agencies led by the US Centers for Disease Control and Prevention have called for states to establish more stringent policies with respect to opioid prescribing.[3] The inherent message is: Decreased prescribing is a principal way to achieve fewer overdose deaths.

Influence of Authoritative Model Policy Templates

Before federal agencies began encouraging states to act in this manner, some states responded to concerns about the use of opioids to treat chronic pain by establishing guidelines for clinicians.

Over the past 2 decades, the Federation of State Medical Boards (FSMB) developed policy templates that contributed to and informed most of the regulatory policy adoption to help guide physicians prescribing for pain management. Beginning with model guidelines issued in 1998,[4] the FSMB attempted to provide physicians with several recommendations considered necessary for safe and appropriate pain care (**Table 1**). These treatment guidelines contain a preamble establishing a context for prescribing, acknowledging pain management as an accepted part of medical practice, and supporting the clinical use of controlled substances, including opioid analgesics, when deemed warranted. The policy further addressed concerns about regulatory scrutiny by assuring physicians that they would not be sanctioned solely for prescribing controlled substances for legitimate medical purposes. The policy template also urged physicians to continually evaluate benefits and risks of treatment and to adopt methods to minimize and, when possible, identify and address diversion-related or abuse-related activities. A multidisciplinary panel of experts composed of representatives from the areas of health care, regulation, law, and policy research, helped draft the model guideline document, which ultimately was formally endorsed by several federal and national organizations. Such organizations included the American Academy of Pain Medicine, the American Medical Association, the American Pain Society, the American Society of Law, Medicine & Ethics, the US Drug Enforcement Administration, the National Association of State Controlled Substances Authorities, and the US Public Health Service, Office of Substance Abuse Treatment.

By 2004, state medical boards were calling for the FSMB to revise the template to ensure that it maintained conformity to current medical opinion and brought additional attention to the undertreatment of pain. As a result, the FSMB updated the model guidelines (now called a *model policy*) to further elaborate boards' expectations related to pain treatment and to clearly define inappropriate practice to include "non-treatment, under-treatment, over-treatment, and continued use of ineffective treatments."[5] The 7 treatment guidelines remained the same, and the description of each was substantively consistent with the previous version, which reinforced the intent to preserve the purpose of the policy template: to improve the quality and consistency of states' health care regulatory board policies. Furthermore, there was a more explicit attempt to convey that the proffered recommendations were not meant to limit or dictate clinical decision making, which was left to a practitioner's discretion (clinical judgment), skills, and expertise. Overall, the 2004 policy reiterated the professional responsibility to assess and treat patients' pain while safeguarding against medication abuse or diversion. Again, the composition of the advisory committee drafting the policy represented similar constituencies as before but was expanded to include law enforcement and patients.

It was not until 2013 that the next revision[6] was issued, taking into account the empirical evidence that had accumulated in the past decade. As such, content from

Table 1
Comparison of Federation of State Medical Boards model guidelines/model policy versions

Model Guidelines (1998)/Model Policy (2004)	Model Policy (2013)
Guidelines	
	Understanding Pain
Evaluation of the Patient	Patient Evaluation and Risk Stratification
Treatment Plan	Development of a Treatment Plan and Goals
Informed Consent and Agreement for Treatment	Informed Consent and Treatment Agreement
	Initiating an Opioid Trial
Periodic Review	Ongoing Monitoring and Adapting the Treatment Plan
	Periodic Drug Testing
Consultation	Consultation and Referral
	Discontinuing Opioid Therapy
Medical Records	Medical Records
Compliance with Controlled Substances Laws and Regulations	Compliance with Controlled Substances Laws and Regulations

the current model policy is more detailed, offering more specific and referenced recommendations to inform treatment decisions and to guide actions to mitigate adverse consequences, all with the same purpose of the previous policies. Although the 7 guidelines from the previous versions are maintained but more thoroughly described, additional guidelines are offered. Further recommendations involve the need to diagnose and treat pain (many of the components of which were originally embedded in the preamble from the first 2 templates) and periodic drug testing (which was expanded from the earlier Informed Consent and Agreement for Treatment section) as well as considerations for initiating and discontinuing opioid therapy. Even though risk/benefit considerations have always been an expected treatment component, this new policy emphasizes this approach in a systematic fashion. The resulting model policy is a considerably more descriptive policy resource for clinicians, which is more in line with the FSMB's *Responsible Opioid Prescribing* books[7,8] that were designed to operationalize the 2004 model policy and facilitate their clinical application. This 2013 template, unlike prior versions, is specific to opioid analgesics used in the treatment of chronic pain; however, the FSMB stresses the applicability of various recommendations to management of other types of pain. Another difference relates to the representation of the expert panel initially invited to develop the policy, which included a variety of federal agencies but did not include legal or patient participation.

Guidelines resulting from these templates do not have the force of law. When issued by regulatory bodies, the policies are meant to provide treatment guidance to physicians (and, in some cases, other prescribers). When offered by expert witnesses and accepted by juries in legal actions, however, they can establish a new standard of practice for opioid prescribing to treat chronic pain.

Guidelines Originating in State Agencies

As state licensing boards began adopting FSMB-based regulatory policies, other state agencies eventually started promulgating clinical practice guidelines that were more explicit in their directions for prescribers. This trend was led by the Washington State Agency Medical Directors' Group, which issued a clinical practice prescribing guideline in 2007; this guideline has been updated several times, most recently in 2015.[9] The Washington guideline was controversial in pain management circles[10] as well as among primary care and other specialty medical groups, but it soon became a model that other states sought to emulate. In 2010, the Washington legislature passed a bill (ESHB 2876) directing the licensing boards regulating all prescribers to draft rules for opioid prescribing.[11] The resulting rules are almost a 1:1 reflection of the treatment language found in the earlier guidelines.

Since that time, most states have established various public policies, including statutes, rules/regulations, and guidelines, seeking to direct opioid prescribers' practices. The specific type of policy has much to do with how closely prescribers need to adhere to them: statutes, rules, and regulations all have the force of law and thus represent mandatory requirements for prescribers. Conversely, guidelines are only advisory in nature and do not represent absolute mandates. As discussed previously, however, even guidelines can have a substantial impact on opioid prescribing practices, because they can be considered in legal and administrative proceedings that place a prescriber's license, livelihood, finances, and freedom at risk. Furthermore, close attention must be paid to the precise language contained in policies: use of the words "shall" or "must" indicate mandatory requirements, whereas use of the word "should" does not, strictly speaking, represent a mandate. Even given this semantic dichotomy, both in terms of providing good patient care and to avoid legal scrutiny, it seems reasonable that any prudent clinician would treat a policy's "shoulds" as "shalls" unless there is an extremely persuasive argument for ignoring the treatment recommendation.

Given the pervasive nature of these directive pain management policies and their ongoing proliferation, it seems that showcasing the content of existing policies may be instructive, for prescribers, advocates, and policymakers. This article presents an examination of the provisions contained in all existing pain management policies that have been issued by state authorities with regulatory oversight over physicians. An overall snapshot of relevant policy provisions is provided, with more in-depth discussion of some of the unique provisions found in various policies.

METHODOLOGY
Policy Collection

A review was conducted of all of the state statutes and regulations in all 50 states and the Washington, DC, related to pharmacists and pharmacy practice and those laws and regulations applicable to physicians, dentists, and optometrists that contain provisions that set forth any type of prescribing and dispensing guidelines pertaining to opioid analgesic medications. That review was accomplished using the Westlaw database by (1) running an initial keyword search in each state and then (2) reviewing the specific state statutes and regulations for any information that may not have come up in the initial keyword search. Using the same methods, the same reviewer accessed and evaluated the medical, dental, and optometry board Web sites for each of the 50 states and Washington, DC, to locate any board policies or guidelines related to prescribing and dispensing.

Policy Evaluation

A content review was then conducted on all identified statutes, regulations (ie, rules), and guidelines (collectively known as *policies*) designed to promote physicians' practices related to pain management. Policies covering other prescribers, such as nurse practitioners, physician assistants, optometrists, dentists, and so forth, were not included in the interest of maintaining a comparable set of policies for review. Two reviewers conducted all evaluations: one reviewer evaluated policies adopted in Alabama through Minnesota (alphabetically), whereas another reviewer was responsible for evaluating policies from the remaining states. Evaluations were completed to identify provisions that set forth recommendations or requirements directing physicians in the prescribing of opioid analgesic medications for the purpose of treating pain. To be eligible for review, the policies must either (1) have the force and effect of law at the time of analysis (statutes and regulations) or (2) be the currently adopted guideline or policy statement of a state medical board or other similar agency responsible for licensing and disciplining physicians. Pain management policies that were issued by entities other than medical boards were not included in this analysis nor were clinical practice guidelines issued by medical associations, professional organizations, and so forth. All policies were evaluated in their entirety, and relevant provisions were sorted into 19 specific categories of provisions commonly found within the policies, plus an "Other" category for unique provisions found in some states' policies. The categories were chosen through a qualitative process that identified common themes with potentially significant clinical implications across policies. These categories comprise the following:

- Statements reassuring physicians regarding, or providing immunity from, disciplinary action for prescribing for a legitimate medical purpose in the usual course of professional practice

- Statements acknowledging or encouraging use of alternatives to opioids
- Statements encouraging a multidisciplinary approach to pain management
- Statements about the need for access to pain relief
- Requirements for patient evaluations
- Threshold opioid doses or durations of treatment
- Urine drug testing (UDT)
- Treatment plans
- Consultation with other clinicians
- Periodic review of patient progress
- Informed consent
- Treatment agreements
- Prescription monitoring programs
- Discussion of risks and benefits
- Control of theft and diversion of opioids
- Qualifications to practice pain management
- Educational requirements
- Distinctions, or lack thereof, between pain resulting from cancer and pain from other causes
- Transitions of care
- Other

A total of 68 policies from 42 states and Washington, DC, were reviewed. **Table 2** contains a concise summary of what types of policy were found in each state, sorted by the 20 types of provisions identified in the review. (The text of each policy, sorted by state and provision, can be found at http://blog.aapainmanage.org/?p=169.)

RESULTS

A substantial portion of the policies that were reviewed are based entirely, or nearly so, on the FSMB model policy documents. Because these policies are redundant due to having the same source, this review focuses on unique provisions in policies developed independently by state agencies.

Statements Acknowledging or Encouraging Use of Alternatives to Opioids

Three state policies stand out in this category of provisions. The most directive of these comes from the Indiana Medical Licensing Board's rule, which requires physicians to use nonopioid options instead of, or in addition to, prescribing opioids where medically appropriate.[12] A less direct statement from the Oregon Medical Board Statements of Philosophy includes the following recommendation: "Opioids are most likely to be successful in reducing pain and restoring function when they are combined with other pain management approaches such as physical therapy and psychological techniques."[13] Both of these statements indicate the desire of these licensing boards to have physicians at least try nonopioid treatments, either instead of or along with opioids in most cases. A slightly different approach comes from the Medical Board of California Medical Guidelines for Prescribing Controlled Substances for Pain, which states, in its section on initiating opioid trials, "Opioid therapy should be presented to the patient as a therapeutic trial or test for a defined period of time (usually no more than 45 days), and with specific evaluation points."[14] Although this does not per se specify that using nonopioid medications and other treatments is desirable, it indicates that the board is concerned about the long-term effectiveness of opioids and anticipates that physicians may need to find alternative methods of treating pain.

Evaluation Requirements

Most policies with evaluation requirement provisions say, in general terms, that physicians must conduct an appropriate evaluation of a patient's painful condition and attempt to determine a diagnosis consistent with the patient's report. Some policies further specify details regarding what needs to be included when evaluating a patient with pain. It is possible that these provisions are included as a response to pill mill practices, in which patient evaluations were extremely minimal, if conducted at all. For example, guidelines from both the Arizona and California medical boards[14,15] are far more detailed. Both guidelines recommend that physicians complete a comprehensive biopsychosocial assessment of a patient's pain and related symptoms and conditions. Guidance also is provided for physicians with respect to assessing a patient's risk of substance abuse and misuse. In both cases, the guidelines list specific assessment instruments that physicians may find useful in carrying out these comprehensive assessments, with California's policy containing appendices with the actual instruments. A regulation with this level of detail would create some risk for physicians who might inadvertently miss 1 or 2 areas in their assessments. Guidelines with such detail, however, more likely serve as helpful resources for physicians.

Urine Drug Testing

Twenty-eight states and the Washington, DC, have policies that discuss UDT as a method of monitoring patients' adherence to prescribed medication regimens and, more often, their use of both licit and illicit nonprescribed drugs. Most of these provisions are general, and most also recommend this practice only for patients who are assessed as high risk for opioid abuse.

A recent trend in pain management practice is to view UDT as a standard monitoring method that is used at various times with all patients at times, with the frequency and perhaps the type of testing determined by a patient's assessed risk. Among the medical board policies with UDT provisions, those from the Arizona, Idaho, Indiana, Kentucky, North Carolina, South Carolina, and West Virginia medical boards[12,15–20] are the most detailed. These policies include features, such as the type of test to be used and the circumstances under which each is most appropriate; reasons for conducting tests; discussion about the differences between medical and forensic UDT; and a variety of other subjects. None of these policies specifies a schedule for testing. In contrast, the Georgia Composite Medical Board's pain management rules[21] specify that physicians must conduct "body fluid analysis (drug screens)" at least 4 times a year if a patient receives Schedule II or III controlled substances for 90 or more consecutive days; an exemption is made for patients with chronic pain from a terminal condition or for patients in a nursing home or hospice.

Given controversies about UDT's cost and potentially fraudulent use,[22,23] it would not be surprising to see medical boards provide more specific guidance to physicians in the coming years.

Consultation with Other Clinicians

Information about referrals to other clinicians is a prevalent phenomenon, with a dozen policies requiring such referrals under some circumstances. Nearly every policy with such a provision mentions the necessity of obtaining a consultation from a mental health specialist if a patient has a mental disorder, and many likewise suggest a consultation with a pain management specialist if a patient's pain is not being adequately managed. Some also recommend consultation with specialists associated

Table 2
Provisions found in state pain management policies

	Requirement			Recommendation		
	Statute	Rule/Regulation	Guideline	Statute	Rule/Regulation	Guideline
Reassurance about prescribing opioids/immunity	AK, CA, MN, MO, ND, NE, NV, NH, NM, OK, OR, RI, WV	MS, NM, OH	OR, SC	—	AL, DE, FL, IA, MA, ME, TX, WA	AZ, DE, DC, ID, IA, KS, KS, MI, MN, NH, OK, OR, VA, VT, WV, WY
Encourages use of alternative treatments	—	DC, IN, KY, NM	—	—	AL, DE, FL, IA, MA, ME, WA, WV	AK, AZ, CA, CO, CT, DE, DC, ID, IA, MI, MN, NC, OH, OK, OR, SC, VA, VT, WY
Encourages multidisciplinary approach	—	—	—	CA, HI	IA, ME, RI	CO, IA, MN, OR, SC
Recognizes need for access to pain relief	—	OK, TX	—	AK, CA, HI, NE, OK	AL, DE, FL, IA, MA, NM, WA	AZ, CA, CT, DE, DC, HI, ID, IA, KS, MI, MN, NC, NH, OK, OR, SC, VA, VT, WV, WY
Evaluation requirements	FL, WV	AK, DE, DC, FL, GA, IN, KY, LA, MS, NJ, NM, OH, OK, OR, RI, TN, TX, WA	NH, OR, SC, WY	—	AL, IA, MA, ME, OK, OR, WA	AK, AZ, CA, CO, CT, DE, DC, HI, ID, IA, KS, MI, MN, NC, NH, OK, VA, VT, WV
Threshold dosages/durations	—	IN, NJ, RI, TN, VT, WA	OH	—	—	CA, CO, SC
UDT	—	DE, DC, FL, GA, IN, KY, LA, NM, OH, TN, TX	—	—	IA, MA, ME, OH, RI	AZ, CA, CO, CT, DE, DC, HI, ID, KS, MI, MN, NC, SC, VA, VT, WV, WY
Treatment plan	FL	DE, DC, FL, KY, LA, MS, NJ, NM, OH, OK, RI, WA	—	—	AL, IA, MA, ME, OK, TX	AK, AZ, CA, CT, DE, DC, HI, ID, KS, MI, MN, NC, NH, SC, VA, VT, WV, WY
Consultation	FL, WV	DE, DC, GA, IN, KY, NJ, NM, OH, RI, WA	—	CA, HI, MN	AL, FL, IA, LA, MA, ME, NJ, OH, OK, RI, TX	AZ, CA, CT, DE, DC, HI, ID, IA, KS, MI, MN, NC, NH, OR, OK, SC, VA, VT, WV

Periodic review	FL	AL, AK, DE, DC, FL, GA, IA, KY, LA, MS, NJ, NM, OH, OK, RI, WA	—	—	MA, ME, OK, RI, TX	AK, AZ, CA, CO, CT, DE, DC, HI, ID, IA, KS, MI, MN, NC, NH, OH, OK, SC, VA, VT, WV, WY
Informed consent	FL	AL, AK, DE, FL, GA, IA, KY, NJ, OH, OR, RI	SC	—	LA, MA, ME, OK, OR, TX	AK, AZ, CA, CT, DE, DC, HI, ID, KS, MI, MN, NC, NH, OH, VA, VT, WV, WY
Treatment agreements	FL	DE, DC, FL, GA, IN, KY, NJ, NM, RI, WA	SC	—	AL, IA, MA, ME, OK, RI, TX, WA	AZ, CA, CO, CT, DE, DC, HI, ID, KS, MI, MN, NC, NH, OH, OK, VA, VT, WV, WY
Prescription monitoring program	WV	IN, KY, MS, NM, RI, TN	SC, VT	—	IA, ME, WA	AZ, CA, CO, DC, ID, OH, OK, OR, VT, WV
Discussion of benefits/risks	FL, MN	DE, DC, FL, IN, IA, KY, NM, OH, OK, OR, RI, WA	—	—	LA, MA, ME, OR, TX	AZ, CA, CO, DE, DC, HI, ID, IA, KS, MI, MN, NC, NH, OK, SC, WV
Theft and diversion control	WV	MS, NJ, NM, OH, RI, TN, WA	OK, VA, VT, WV, WY	—	AL, FL, IA, MA, ME	AK, CA, CO, CT, DE, DC, HI, ID, IA, KS, MN, NC, OK, SC, WV
Qualifications	WV	GA, MA, MS, OH, RI, TN, WA	—	—	—	—
Education	MI, NM, SC	IA, KY, MA, MS, NM, OH, RI, TN, TX	VT	—	OH, WA	—
Cancer/noncancer distinction	NM	IN, KY, LA, MS, NM, OH, WA	RI, VT	—	SC	AZ, CA, CO, DC, DE, ID, NC, OK, WV
Transition of care	—	GA, RI	—	—	—	NC, OK, SC, VA, VT, WV
Other	MO, ND, NH	GA, IN, NJ, NM, OH, OK, TN, WA	KS, NH, SC	AK, CA, NE, OK	FL, ME, TX, WA	AK, CA, CO, NC, OK, OR, SC, VA, VT, WV, WY

with the diagnosed or suspected cause of a patient's pain (eg, a rheumatologist if a patient is thought to have arthritis).

As with other provisions, several policies are more specific in their consultation recommendations. The South Carolina Boards of Medical Examiners, Dentistry, and Nursing, in their joint pain management guideline,[19(p4)] suggest consultation with "specialists in psychology, psychiatry, and addiction management if possible...when opioids are identified as the best treatment option for complex or high-risk patients." Neither "complex" nor "high-risk" is defined, and such ambiguity may muddle practitioners' interpretations of this recommendation.

The Rhode Island Department of Health's pain management rules[24] suggest referrals to "other professionals such as chiropractors, acupuncturists, behavioral health providers, [and] physical therapists" and later state that physicians are required to document consideration of a consultation with a pain management specialist if a patient's prescribed dose meets or exceeds 120 mg in oral morphine equivalents per day (MEDs).

Finally, rules promulgated by the Washington State Medical Quality Assurance Commission mandate a consultation when adult patients reach a threshold of 120 mg oral MEDs, unless certain exceptions are met.[25] Those exceptions include situations in which (1) a patient's dose is above that threshold, but the patient's pain and function are stable; (2) a patient's dose is being tapered but still above the threshold; and (3) the prescribing physician meets the rule's qualification criteria for a pain management specialist.

Many policies recommend consultation for patients who are deemed at high risk of medication abuse, misuse, or diversion. Although it is easy to surmise that a mental health clinician specializing in drug abuse and addiction might be a good referral for a patient who might engage in abuse or misuse, it is not clear what kind of medical professional is best consulted to help a patient avoid engaging in diversion.

Periodic Review

Most policies contain provisions regarding the need for physicians to see patients with pain regularly for follow-up appointments to assess progress toward treatment goals and to evaluate for the occurrence of adverse drug-related events, including substance abuse or addiction. Two regulatory policies, however, contain unique language that warrants special mention.

The Alaska State Medical Board's guideline[26(p1)] advises that regular appointments are fundamental but then adds a totally unique condition, stating, "[d]rug holidays to evaluate for symptom recurrence or withdrawal are important." The concept of drug holidays is one that has fallen out of favor in pain management and is completely absent from all the other guidelines reviewed in this article.

The other policy worthy of special mention is the Georgia Composite Medical Board's rules for pain management.[21] Patients prescribed Schedule II or III controlled substances for 90 consecutive days to treat chronic pain are mandated to have a written treatment agreement that requires patients to have a clinical visit at least once every 3 months while undergoing treatment of pain. Recall that this rule also mandates UDT at 3-month intervals, suggesting that the Georgia Board was trying to communicate that physicians should monitor such patients closely and regularly.

Informed Consent

Thirty-two states and the Washington, DC, have policies discussing informed consent, with a slight preference for policies that recommend, rather than require, this element in a patient's treatment. Most of these requirements and recommendations are straightforward, mandating or suggesting that patients should give formal informed consent to treatment with opioids or with controlled substances in general. Provisions from 2 state medical boards warrant further consideration due to their unique characteristics.

Arkansas rules governing pain treatment[27] consider a physician who prescribes Schedule II–V controlled substances, excluding tramadol, for more than 6 months to treat pain not associated with "malignant or terminal illness" as guilty of gross negligence or ignorant malpractice unless several conditions are met. One of these conditions is as follows: "The physician will obtain written informed consent from those patients he or she is concerned may abuse controlled substances..." This requirement is curious, in part because it applies only to those patients considered high risk for substance abuse and partly because the goal of such informed consent is not fully explained. It also is unclear whether having a patient acknowledge the risk of substance abuse is effective in preventing that eventuality from occurring.

The second unique provision is contained in the Medical Board of California's guidelines.[14(p11)] In addition to counseling patients to obtain a recommended informed consent, physicians are advised to instruct patients and possibly family members on "safe ways to store and dispose of medications." Although discussions of safe storage and disposal have grown in favor in recent years, their inclusion in informed consent documentation is uniquely anticipated by this policy.

Treatment Agreements

Treatment agreements (sometimes known by the misnomers *opioid contracts* or *pain contracts*) are frequently promoted as tools to minimize the risk of opioid misuse, abuse, and diversion, despite the absence of consistent evidence that they actually achieve this objective.[28] Thirty-seven policies reviewed for this report contain provisions related to these agreements. Most policies specify that agreements should contain statements about what a patient can and cannot do with respect to pain medications, with various consequences specified for violations of those terms of the agreements. Some policies also include recommendations regarding physician responsibility to patients (eg, that there is another prescriber available to provide coverage if the physician is not available). For more in-depth information about the current status of treatment agreements in pain management, readers are referred to a policy brief published by the Pain Action Alliance to Implement a National Strategy.[29]

Among the policies reviewed, Iowa's Board of Medicine Standards of Practice and Principles of Medical Ethics[30] are notable for its strong recommendation: "A physician prescribing controlled substances to a patient for more than 90 days to treat chronic pain should use a written agreement if the patient is deemed high-risk with respect to drug abuse or diversion; if the physician decides not to use an agreement, he or she must document the reasons for such a decision." Similarly, the Kentucky Board of Medical Licensure's standards for prescribing and dispensing controlled substances[17] require the use of a prescribing agreement, which "meets professional standards" if a physician determines a risk that a patient may illegally divert a controlled substance but nevertheless decides to continue prescribing. Such a mandate can lead to physician confusion about the appropriate treatment agreement template, because currently there are no established professional standards for such prescribing agreements.

Qualifications of Physicians

Nine policies contain qualification standards for practitioners providing pain management services, including in certain types of medical settings. Of these, only West Virginia[31] has standards in statute, whereas the rest are found in regula-tions. Each of these policies, with the exception of the one from Massachusetts,[32] provides that a physician with a board certification or certificate of subspecializa-tion in pain medicine meets the criteria to

- Work in a pain management clinic (Georgia and Mississippi)[21,33]
- Own a pain management clinic (West Virginia and Ohio)[31,34]
- Be the medical director of a pain management clinic (Tennessee)[35]
- Be designated a pain medicine specialist under the state's rules (Rhode Island and Washington)[24,25]

Some policies also allow alternative paths to these endpoints, such as eligibility for the designated certifications, completion of specific training programs, or completion of a certain amount and type of continuing medical education. In Massachusetts, the law[32] specifies that all physicians must complete 3 hours of pain management continuing medical education to obtain or renew a medical license.

Threshold Doses and Durations

Perhaps the most controversial provision to appear in pain management policies has been the use of threshold doses for opioid analgesics. Under this standard, if a patient's prescribed opioid analgesic dose meets or exceeds the designated threshold, certain actions must occur. A dosage threshold was first established in the Washington State Agency Medical Directors' Group guideline (discussed previously)[9] and then subsequently established in prescribers' regulations. It seems that the intent of most of these regulatory provisions is to help ensure that physicians prescribe high-dose opioids to their patients only when there is evidence that this treatment is effective and that benefits outweigh harms. It is likely, though, that some prescribers may treat these threshold doses as de facto ceiling doses, whereas others may cease prescribing opioids altogether due to fearing sanction for inadver-tently violating the rules. Additional concerns about these policies are outlined in a recent article by Ziegler.[36]

Policies with threshold dose provisions run the gamut from simple and minimally directive to complicated and extraordinarily detailed. Representing the simplest and least burdensome versions, California[14] recommends that caution should be exercised at doses exceeding 80 mg MEDs and that a pain specialist consultation should be considered, whereas Colorado[37] acknowledges that doses exceeding 120 mg MEDs are more dangerous, so that additional safeguards should be used, and consultation or referral should be considered. Rules from Rhode Island[24] are similarly simple, specifying that at 120 mg MEDs, physicians must consider a referral to a pain management specialist and document that consideration in a patient's record.

Shifting from an emphasis on dose thresholds to duration thresholds, Vermont's rules[38] mandate that physicians tell patients that, when starting treatment with opioid analgesics, that treatment is on a trial basis. The rules recommend that the trial last no longer than 90 days, after which opioid treatment should be continued only if the patient is evaluated and found to be benefitting from the treatment.

Tennessee and New Jersey both have rules requiring that physicians justify pre-scribing more than certain quantities of medication. In Tennessee,[35] physicians must document the reason for prescribing more than a 72-hour supply of opioids but only if those physicians are working in a licensed pain management clinic; those working in other settings, including primary care practices, are not subject to this requirement. New Jersey has developed regulations requiring that physicians justify prescribing both on quantity of medication and duration of treatment.[39] In New Jersey, physicians are prohibited from writing prescriptions for more than 120 dosage units or a 30-day supply of an opioid unless certain criteria are met. To exceed 120 dosage units, physicians must document that there is an individualized treatment plan with measurable objectives for that treatment. Correspondingly, to exceed a 30-day supply, the medication must be administered through an implanted pump or the prescription must be part of a prescription series that follows federal prescribing rules.

More detailed guidance is provided by policies in Washington, Indiana, Ohio, and South Carolina. In Washington,[25] as discussed previously, patients whose opioid prescriptions meet or exceed 120 mg MEDs are required to be referred for consultation with a pain management specialist, provided their pain and function are not stable and their opioid dose is not being tapered. Indiana requires that when a patient's daily opioid dose meets or exceeds 60 mg MEDs, the physician must conduct a face-to-face re-evaluation of the patient, consider a referral to a pain management specialist, and develop a new treatment plan with specified outcome goals. Ohio's policy[40] mandates that several things happen if a patient is prescribed 80 mg MEDs or more for 3 consecutive months for treatment of nonterminal pain. When this happens, the physician must re-establish informed consent, document a complete assessment of the patient's pain and functioning, document progress toward goals, check the state prescription monitoring program database, consider establishing a treatment agreement with the patient, consider a consultation with a specialist relevant to the type of pain experienced by the patient, and perform a substance abuse assessment. Finally, South Carolina[19] has essentially adopted Ohio's provisions but has placed them in a voluntary guideline rather than in a mandatory rule.

In addition to currently adopted regulatory policies, several states have introduced legislation to establish various threshold doses, with assorted actions required after reaching that dose. Several factors should be acknowledged by policymakers considering such policies, including

1. There are, as yet, no outcome data demonstrating that these threshold policies are effective in reducing overdose deaths and opioid abuse/misuse/diversion.
2. Similarly, further evidence is necessary to determine the extent that people with a legitimate medical need for opioids are not harmed by these policies.
3. There is a shortage of qualified pain management specialists available to receive the consultations that are recommended or required under these policies, as demonstrated by surveys in Washington.[41]

Additionally, there are numerous scientific challenges associated with determining equianalgesic dosing and interindividual differences in response to a given opioid dose. These individual differences mean that clinicians need to use an individualized approach to treatment, because each patient presents a unique combination of positive and negative responses to any given dose of any given opioid. This ability to exercise appropriate clinical flexibility can be severely limited if policies mandate certain actions at certain doses. For some patients, those actions are clinically appropriate at those doses (and perhaps even before reaching those doses), whereas for others, the mandated or recommended course of action represents an unnecessary intrusion into the physician-patient relationship. More work needs to be done to refine these provisions and to prove that they provide an appropriate balance of positive intended versus negative unintended consequences.

DISCUSSION

The rapid proliferation of state policies related to the practice of pain medicine has been remarkable. With most states having at least 1 policy and several having multiple policies, it is time for state agencies administering these policies to team with academic researchers to determine the effectiveness of such policies. This determination should examine both the intended effects (reductions in opioid misuse, abuse, addiction, and related overdose) and the unintended effects (restriction of access for patients with a legitimate medical need and demonstrated benefit from using opioids). Such an examination should provide policymakers with guidance on how policies can be modified to maximize their intended benefits and minimize their unintended harms—much as the policies seek to do for pain treatment involving opioid analgesics. In a sense, what is really needed is more evidence to guide both the evidence-based practice of pain management and evidence-based public policy development.

ACKNOWLEDGMENTS

The authors wish to acknowledge the significant contribution of Heather Gray, JD. Ms Gray maintains a database of state pain policies and provided that database as the starting point for this article's analysis. Her significant contribution is greatly appreciated.

REFERENCES

1. US Centers for Disease Control and Prevention. Injury prevention and control: prescription drug overdose. Data overview. 2015. Available at: http://www.cdc.gov/drugoverdose/data/index.html. Accessed November 16, 2015.
2. US Centers for Disease Control and Prevention. Vital signs: overdoses of prescription opioid pain relievers—United States, 1999-2008. MMWR Morb Mortal Wkly Rep 2011;60(43):1487–92.
3. US Centers for Disease Control and Prevention. What states need to know about the epidemic. 2015. Available at: http://www.cdc.gov/drugoverdose/epidemic/states.html. Accessed November 16, 2015.
4. Federation of State Medical Boards (FSMB). Model guidelines for the use of controlled substances for the treatment of pain. Washington, DC: The Federation; 1998.
5. Federation of State Medical Boards (FSMB). Model policy for the use of controlled substances for the treatment of pain. Washington, DC: The Federation; 2004.
6. Federation of State Medical Boards (FSMB). Model policy for the use of opioid analgesics in the treatment of pain. Washington, DC: The Federation; 2013.
7. Fishman SM. Responsible opioid prescribing: a clinician's guide. Washington, DC: The Federation of State Medical Boards (FSMB); 2007.
8. Fishman SM. Responsible opioid prescribing: a clinician's guide. 2nd edition. Washington, DC: The Federation of State Medical Boards (FSMB); 2014.
9. Washington State Agency Medical Directors' Group. Interagency guideline on prescribing opioids for pain. 2015. Available at: http://www.agencymeddirectors.wa.gov/Files/2015AMDGOpioidGuideline.pdf. Accessed November 16, 2015.
10. Ostrom CM, Williams LC. New state pain-medication law has doctors and patients nervous. Seattle Times 2010. Available at: http://www.seattletimes.com/seattle-news/new-state-pain-medication-law-has-doctors-and-patients-nervous/. Accessed November 16, 2015.

11. State of Washington. Engrossed substitute house bill 2876: pain management—adoption of rules. 2010. Available at: http://apps.leg.wa.gov/documents/billdocs/2009-10/Pdf/Bills/Session%20Laws/House/2876-S.SL.pdf. Accessed November 16, 2015.
12. Indiana Code § 844-5-6-4; 2015.
13. Oregon Medical Board. Statements of philosophy: pain management. 2013. Available at: http://www.oregon.gov/omb/board/philosophy/Pages/Pain-Management.aspx. Accessed November 16, 2015.
14. Medical Board of California. Guidelines for prescribing controlled substances for pain. 2014. Available at: http://www.mbc.ca.gov/licensees/prescribing/pain_guidelines.pdf. Accessed November 16, 2014.
15. Arizona Medical Board. Reference for physicians on the use of opioid analgesics in the treatment of chronic pain, in the office setting. 2014. Available at: http://www.azdhs.gov/documents/audiences/clinicians/clinical-guidelines-recommendations/prescribing-guidelines/141121-opiod.pdf. Accessed November 16, 2015.
16. Idaho Medical Board. Policy for the use of opioid analgesics in the treatment of chronic pain. 2013. Available at: https://c.ymcdn.com/sites/www.idahopa.org/resource/resmgr/Docs/ModelPolicyUseofOpioidAnalge.pdf. Accessed November 16, 2015.
17. Kentucky Rev. Stat. Ann. § 201.9–260.
18. North Carolina Medical Board. Policy for the use of opiates for the treatment of pain. 2014. Available at: http://www.ncmedboard.org/images/uploads/other_pdfs/Policy_for_the_Use_of_Opiates_for_the_Treatment_of_Pain_June_4_2014.pdf. Accessed November 16, 2015.
19. South Carolina Board of Medical Examiners. Joint revised pain management guidelines approved by the South Carolina boards of medical examiners, dentistry, and nursing. 2014. Available at: http://www.llr.state.sc.us/POL/Medical/PDF/Joint_Revised_Pain_Management_Guidelines.pdf. Accessed November 16, 2015.
20. West Virginia Board of Medicine. Policy for the use of opioid analgesics in the treatment of chronic pain. 2013. Available at: https://wvbom.wv.gov/download_resource.asp?id=9. Accessed November 16, 2015.
21. Georgia Code Ann. § 360-3-.06.
22. Weaver C, Mathews AW. Doctors cash in on drug tests for seniors, and Medicare pays the bill. Wall Street Journal 2014. Available at: http://www.wsj.com/articles/doctors-cash-in-on-drug-tests-for-seniors-and-medicare-pays-the-bill-1415676782. Accessed November 16, 2014.
23. Weaver C, Mathews AW. Lab nears settlement over pricey Medicare drug tests. Wall Street Journal 2015. Available at: http://www.wsj.com/articles/lab-nears-settlementover-pricey-medicare-drug-tests-1434326131. Accessed November 16, 2015.
24. 6 Rhode Island Gen. Laws Ann. § 31-2-6:3.9.
25. Washington Admin. Code § 246-919-860.
26. Alaska State Medical Board. Board issued guidelines: prescribing controlled substances. 1997. Available at: https://www.commerce.alaska.gov/web/portals/5/pub/MED_Guide_Prescribing_Controlled_Substances.pdf. Accessed November 16, 2015.
27. Arkansas State Medical Board. Regulation No. 2. 2012. Available at: http://www.armedicalboard.org/professionals/pdf/mpa.pdf. Accessed November 16, 2015.
28. Starrels JL, Becker WC, Alford DP, et al. Systematic review: treatment agreements and urine drug testing to reduce opioid misuse in patients with chronic pain. Ann Intern Med 2010;152:712–20.

29. Payne R, Twillman R. Policy brief: opioid treatment agreements or "contracts": proceed with caution. 2014. Available at: http://www.painsproject.org/wp/wp-content/uploads/2014/05/pain-policy-issue4-e-mailable.pdf. Accessed November 16, 2015.

30. Iowa Admin. Code. § 653–13.2(148,272C): Standards of practice—appropriate pain management.

31. West Virginia Code § 16-5H-4.

32. Massachusetts 243 CMR § 2.02.

33. Mississippi Code Ann. § 30-17-2640:1.15.

34. Ohio Admin. Code § 4731-29-01.

35. Tennessee Department of Health Rules, Chapter 1200-34-01.

36. Ziegler SJ. The proliferation of dosage thresholds in opioid prescribing policies and their potential to increase pain and opioid-related mortality. Pain Med 2015;16(10):1851–6.

37. Colorado Department of Regulatory Agencies. Policy for prescribing and dispensing opioids. 2014. Available at: https://drive.google.com/file/d/0B-K5D hxXxJZbd01vVXdTTkIZLVU/view. Accessed November 16, 2015.

38. Vermont Board of Medical Practice. Policy on the use of opioid analgesics in the treatment of chronic pain. 2014. Available at: http://healthvermont.gov/hc/med_board/documents/opioid_pain_treatment_policy.pdf. Accessed November 16, 2015.

39. New Jersey Admin. Code § 13:35–7.6.

40. State Medical Board of Ohio. Guidelines for prescribing opioids for the treatment of chronic, non-terminal pain. 2013. Available at: http://www.opioidprescribing.ohio.gov/PDF/oarrs/Print_Prescribing_Guidelinesfor%20.pdf. Accessed November 16, 2015.

41. Franklin GM, Fulton-Kehoe D, Turner JA, et al. Changes in opioid prescribing for chronic pain in Washington state. J Am Board Fam Med 2013;26(4):394–400.

Index

Note: Page numbers of article titles are in **boldface** type.

A

Ablative therapies, image-guided percutaneous, for cancer pain, 334–336
    cryoablation, 334–335
    radiofrequency ablation, 334
Abuse-deterrent technology, chronic pain and opioids, 346
Acetaminophen, for acute pain in the emergency department, 274–275
Acute pain, management in the emergency department, 272–277
    acetaminophen, 273–274
    channels/enzymes/receptors targeted analgesia concept, 276–277, 278–279
    ketamine, 274
    local anesthetics, 275–276
    nitrous oxide, 276
    NSAIDs, 273
    opioids, 272–273
  managing opioid-tolerant patients in the perioperative surgical home, **287–301**
    definitions, 288–289
      opioid tolerance, 289
      opioid-induced hyperalgesia, 289
      opioids, 288
      perioperative surgical home concept, 288
    intraoperative management, 292–294
      dexmedetomidine, 294
      ketamine, 292–293
      lidocaine infusions, 293
      regional anesthesia and analgesia, 293
    postoperative management, 294–295
      multimodal approach to, 294–295
      oral analgesics and restarting home medications, 295
    preoperative assessment, 289–292
    special considerations for opioid addiction therapy, 295–298
      acute pain management services in, 297–298
      buprenorphine, 296–297
      naltrexone, 297
Acute pain management service, in the perioperative surgical home, 297–298
Addiction therapy, opioid, special perioperative considerations for patients on, 295–297
Affordable Care Act, using chronic pain outcomes data to improve outcomes, 398–399
    bundled payment for care improvement services, 398–399
    chronic care management services, 399
American Academy of Pain Medicine, guidelines for opioid use in chronic pain, 348–350
American Pain Society, guidelines for opioid use in chronic pain, 348–350
Amputation, phantom limb pain after, 305
Analgesia. *See* Pain management.

Anesthesiology Clin 34 (2016) 425–437
http://dx.doi.org/10.1016/S1932-2275(16)30019-2
1932-2275/16/$ – see front matter
anesthesiology.theclinics.com

Anticonvulsants, for sleep disturbance in patients with chronic pain, 388
Antidepressants, for sleep disturbance in patients with chronic pain, 386–388
Antipsychotics, for sleep disturbance in patients with chronic pain, 388

B

Benzodiazepine receptor agonists, for sleep disturbance in patients with
    chronic pain, 385–386
Brain-based therapies, for chronic pain, role of neuroimaging in, **255–269**
Breast surgery, persistent postsurgical pain after, 304
Buprenorphine, for opioid addiction therapy, perioperative management of
    patients on, 296–297

C

Canadian National Opioid Use Guideline Group, guidelines for opioid use in
    chronic pain, 348–350
Cancer pain, interventional treatments for, **317–339**
        image-guided percutaneous tumor ablation, 334–336
            cryoablation, 334–335
            radiofrequency ablation, 334
        intrathecal drug delivery, 318–322
            complications of, 320, 321
            efficacy of, 320–322
            indications, 318
            methods of, 318–320
            ongoing oncologic care and, 322
            pharmacologic options, 318, 319
        neurolytic plexus blocks, 324–334
            celiac plexus neurolysis, 326–328
            ganglion impar neurolysis, 330–331
            intercostal neurolysis, 331–332
            of the extremities, 334
            peripheral nerve neurolytic blockade, 331
            superior hypogastric plexus neurolysis, 328–329
            trigeminal neurolysis, 332–334
        others, 336
            intrathecal neurolysis, 336
            neurosurgical procedures, 336
            spinal cord stimulation, 336
        vertebral augmentation, 324
            complications, 324
            contraindications, 324
            indications, 324
            outcomes, 324
Celiac plexus neurolysis, for cancer pain, 326–328
Centers for Medicare and Medicaid Services (CMS), outcomes and opioid
    prescription programs, 399–401
Channels/enzymes/receptors targeted analgesia (CERTA), for acute pain in
    the emergency department, 276–277, 278–279
Chronic care management services, 399

Chronic pain, and the opioid conundrum, **341–355**
    abuse deterrent technology, 346
    background, 342–344
        on chronic pain, 342–343
        on opioid-related death, misuse, abuse, addiction, 343–344
    lessons learned from history, 341–342
    opioid effectiveness data, 344–345
    principles of practice, 348–350
        guidelines from professional medical societies, 348–350
    problem with payer policies, 346
    regulatory considerations, 347–348
        FDA labeling changes, 348
        rescheduling of hydrocodone, 348
        risk evaluation and mitigation strategy programs, 347
        upper dose limits, 347
    research needed, 346
  imaging of, **255–269**
    anatomical and functional substrates, 256–258
    findings, 258–263
        limitations of neuroimaging research, 261–263
        multivariate analysis of imaging data, 261
        network-based changes in brain function, 260–261
        regional changes in brain function, 259–260
        regional changes in brain structure, 258–259
  management in the emergency department, 277, 280
  persistent postsurgical pain, **303–315**
    analgesia for prevention of, 309–311
        gabapentin, 309–310
        ketamine, 310
        multimodal, 311
        NSAIDs, 309
        pregabalin, 310
        regional anesthesia/neuroaxial anesthesia, 310–311
    common surgical procedures associated with, 304–305
        breast surgery, 304
        postamputation phantom limb pain, 305
        thoracic surgery, 304–305
    genetics/epigenetics of, 306–307
    mechanisms for development of, 305–306
    risk factors for development of, 307–309
  sleep disturbance in patients with, **379–393**
    assessment of, 381–382
    nonpharmacologic interventions, 382–383
    pharmacotherapy, 383–389
        anticonvulsants, 388
        antidepressants, 386–388
        antipsychotics, 388
        benzodiazepine receptor agonists, 385–386
        nonbenzodiazepine benzodiazepine receptor agonists, 386
        opioid analgesics, 383–385
        over the counter medications, 388–389

Chronic (*continued*)
using outcomes data to improve outcomes with, **395–408**
Affordable Care Act, 398–399
bundled payment for care improvement services, 398–399
chronic care management services, 399
Centers for Medicare and Medicaid Services outcomes and opioid prescription programs, 399–401
health care economics, 396–397
integrating mobile technology, 405–406
integration into electronic health records, 404–405
patient-reported outcome measures, 401
tracking pain outcomes on a national level, 397–398
Tri-Institutional Pain Registry, 401–404
utilizing data to improve efficiency and quality, 397
Chronification, of pain in veterans, prevention and reversal of, 360–362
Cognitive behavior therapy, for sleep disturbance in patients with chronic pain, 382
combined treatment of pain and sleep, 383
for insomnia, 382–383
for pain, 382
Cryoablation, for cancer pain, 334–335

D

Dexmedetomidine, intraoperative, in opioid-tolerant patients, 294
Dosage thresholds, for opioids, state policies on, 420–421

E

Economics, of health care, 396–397
Electronic health records, integration of patient-reported outcomes into, 404–405
Emergency department, pain management in, **271–285**
acute pain, 272–277
acetaminophen, 273–274
channels/enzymes/receptors targeted analgesia concept, 276–277
ketamine, 274
local anesthetics, 275–276
nitrous oxide, 276
NSAIDs, 273
opioids, 272–273
chronic pain, 277–280
Epigenetics, of persistent postsurgical pain, 306–307

F

Food and Drug Administration (FDA), opioid labeling changes, 348

G

Gabapentin, for prevention of persistent postsurgical pain, 309–310
Ganglion impar neurolysis, for cancer pain, 330–331
Genetics, of persistent postsurgical pain, 306–307
Guidelines, for opioid use in chronic pain, 348–350

H

Hydrocodone, rescheduling of, 348
Hyperalgesia, opioid-induced, 289

I

Imaging, of chronic pain, **255–269**
        anatomical and functional substrates, 256–258
        findings, 258–263
            limitations of neuroimaging research, 261–263
            multivariate analysis of imaging data, 261
            network-based changes in brain function, 260–261
            regional changes in brain function, 259–260
            regional changes in brain structure, 258–259
Informed consent, state policies on, 418–419
Intercostal neurolysis, for cancer pain, 331–332
Intranasal analgesia, of opioids, for acute pain in the emergency department, 273
Intrathecal drug delivery, for cancer pain, 318–322
        complications of, 320, 321
        efficacy of, 320–322
        indications, 318
        methods of, 318–320
        ongoing oncologic care and, 322
        pharmacologic options, 318, 319
Intrathecal neurolysis, for cancer pain, 336

J

Joint Pain Education Project, from the VA and Dept. of Defense, 368

K

Ketamine, for acute pain in the emergency department, 275
    for prevention of persistent postsurgical pain, 310
    intraoperative, in opioid-tolerant patients, 292–293

L

Lidocaine infusions, intraoperative, in opioid-tolerant patients, 293–294
Local anesthetics, for acute pain in the emergency department, 275–276
        intra-articular, 276
        regional (ultrasound-guided nerve blocks), 275–276
        systemic (intravenous), 276
        topical, 275

M

Magnetic resonance imaging, resting state function, of brain function, 260–261
Military personnel. *See also* Veterans.
pain in, 359–360

Mobile technology, integration of, into chronic pain management and outcomes, 405–406

Multimodal analgesia, for postoperative analgesia in opioid-tolerant patients, 294–295

    for prevention of persistent postsurgical pain, 311

Multivariate pattern analysis, of neuroimaging data, 261

N

Naltrexone, for opioid addiction therapy, perioperative management of patients on, 297

Nebulized analgesia, of opioids, for acute pain in the emergency department, 273

Neuroaxial anesthesia, for prevention of persistent postsurgical pain, 310–311

Neuroimaging, of chronic pain, **255–269**

    anatomical and functional substrates, 256–258

    findings, 258–263

        limitations of research on, 261–263

        multivariate analysis of imaging data, 261

        network-based changes in brain function, 260–261

        regional changes in brain function, 259–260

        regional changes in brain structure, 258–259

Neurolytic plexus blocks, for cancer pain, 324–334

    celiac plexus neurolysis, 326–328

    ganglion impar neurolysis, 330–331

    intercostal neurolysis, 331–332

    of the extremities, 334

    peripheral nerve neurolytic blockade, 331

    superior hypogastric plexus neurolysis, 328–329

    trigeminal neurolysis, 332–334

Neurosurgical procedures, for cancer pain, 336

Nitrous oxide, for acute pain in the emergency department, 276

Nonsteroidal antiinflammatory drugs (NSAIDs), for acute pain in the emergency department, 274

    for prevention of persistent postsurgical pain, 309

Nursing, Pain Management Nursing Group, from the VA and Dept. of Defense, 371

O

Opioid addiction therapy, special perioperative considerations for patients on, 295–297

    buprenorphine, 296–297

    naltrexone, 297

Opioid Safety Initiative, from the VA and Dept. of Defense, 370–371

Opioid-tolerant patients, management in the perioperative surgical home, **287–301**

    definitions, 288–289

        opioid tolerance, 289

        opioid-induced hyperalgesia, 289

        opioids, 288

        perioperative surgical home concept, 288

    intraoperative management, 292–294

        dexmedetomidine, 294

            ketamine, 292–293
            lidocaine infusions, 293
            regional anesthesia and analgesia, 293
        postoperative management, 294–295
            multimodal approach to, 294–295
            oral analgesics and restarting home medications, 295
        preoperative assessment, 289–292
        special considerations for opioid addiction therapy, 295–298
            acute pain management services in, 297–298
            buprenorphine, 296–297
            naltrexone, 297
Opioids, chronic pain and the conundrum with, **341–355**
        abuse deterrent technology, 346
        background, 342–344
            on chronic pain, 342–343
            on opioid-related death, misuse, abuse, addiction, 343–344
        lessons learned from history, 341–342
        opioid effectiveness data, 344–345
        principles of practice, 348–350
            guidelines from professional medical societies, 348–350
        problem with payer policies, 346
        regulatory considerations, 347–348
            FDA labeling changes, 348
            rescheduling of hydrocodone, 348
            risk evaluation and mitigation strategy programs, 347
            upper dose limits, 347
        research needed, 346
    dosage thresholds for, state policies on, 420–421
    for acute pain in the emergency department, 272–273
        nebulized/intranasal analgesia, 273
        parenteral (intravenous) dosing, 272–273
        patient-controlled analgesia, 273
    for sleep disturbance in patients with chronic pain, 383–385
    management of opioid-tolerant patients in perioperative surgical home,
        287–301
    state policies on use of alternatives to, 414
Outcomes data, on chronic pain, use of to improve outcomes, **395–408**
        Affordable Care Act, 398–399
            bundled payment for care improvement services, 398–399
            chronic care management services, 399
        Centers for Medicare and Medicaid Services outcomes and opioid
            prescription programs, 399–401
        health care economics, 396–397
        integrating mobile technology, 405–406
        integration into electronic health records, 404–405
        patient-reported outcome measures, 401
        tracking pain outcomes on a national level, 397–398
        Tri-Institutional Pain Registry, 401–404
        utilizing data to improve efficiency and quality, 397
Over-the-counter medications, for sleep disturbance in patients with chronic pain,
    388–389

P

Pain management, 255–424
    chronic pain and the opioid conundrum, **341–355**
        abuse deterrent technology, 346
        background, 342–344
            on chronic pain, 342–343
            on opioid-related death, misuse, abuse, addiction, 343–344
        lessons learned from history, 341–342
        opioid effectiveness data, 344–345
        principles of practice, 348–350
            guidelines from professional medical societies, 348–350
        problem with payer policies, 346
        regulatory considerations, 347–348
            FDA labeling changes, 348
            rescheduling of hydrocodone, 348
            risk evaluation and mitigation strategy programs, 347
            upper dose limits, 347
        research needed, 346
    imaging pain, **255–269**
        anatomical and functional substrates, 256–258
        findings, 258–263
            limitations of chronic pain neuroimaging research, 261–263
            multivariate analysis of imaging data, 261
            network-based changes in brain function, 260–261
            regional changes in brain function, 259–260
            regional changes in brain structure, 258–259
    in the emergency department, **271–285**
        acute pain, 272–277
            acetaminophen, 273–274
            channels/enzymes/receptors targeted analgesia concept, 276–277, 278–279
            ketamine, 274
            local anesthetics, 275–276
            nitrous oxide, 276
            NSAIDs, 273
            opioids, 272–273
        chronic pain, 277, 280
    in the veteran population, **357–378**
        pain as a public health problem, 357–359
        pain in military personnel and veterans, 359–360
        prevention and reversal of pain chronification, 360–362
        providing education and training, 368–371
        stepped-care approach, 365–368
        structural challenges, 362–365
        VA pain research, 372
    interventional treatments for cancer pain, **317–339**
        image-guided percutaneous tumor ablation, 334–336
            cryoablation, 334–335
            radiofrequency ablation, 334
        intrathecal drug delivery, 318–322
            complications of, 320, 321

efficacy of, 320–322
indications, 318
methods of, 318–320
ongoing oncologic care and, 322
pharmacologic options, 318, 319
neurolytic plexus blocks, 324–334
celiac plexus neurolysis, 326–328
ganglion impar neurolysis, 330–331
intercostal neurolysis, 331–332
of the extremities, 334
peripheral nerve neurolytic blockade, 331
superior hypogastric plexus neurolysis, 328–329
trigeminal neurolysis, 332–334
others, 336
intrathecal neurolysis, 336
neurosurgical procedures, 336
spinal cord stimulation, 336
vertebral augmentation, complications, 324
contraindications, 324
indications, 324
outcomes, 324
of opioid-tolerant patients in the perioperative surgical home, **287–301**
definitions, 288–289
opioid tolerance, 289
opioid-induced hyperalgesia, 289
opioids, 288
perioperative surgical home concept, 288
intraoperative management, 292–294
dexmedetomidine, 294
ketamine, 292–293
lidocaine infusions, 293
regional anesthesia and analgesia, 293
postoperative management, 294–295
multimodal approach to, 294–295
oral analgesics and restarting home medications, 295
preoperative assessment, 289–292
special considerations for opioid addiction therapy, 295–298
acute pain management services in, 297–298
buprenorphine, 296–297
naltrexone, 297
persistent postsurgical pain, **303–315**
analgesia for prevention of, 309–311
common surgical procedures associated with, 304–305
breast surgery, 304
postamputation phantom limb pain, 305
thoracic surgery, 304–305
genetics/epigenetics of, 306–307
mechanisms for development of, 305–306
risk factors for development of, 307–309
sleep disturbance in patients with chronic pain, **379–393**
assessment of, 381–382

Pain (*continued*)
    nonpharmacologic interventions, 382–383
    pharmacotherapy, 383–389
   state policies regulating practice of, **409–424**
    authoritative model policy templates, 410–411
    guidelines originating in state agencies, 412–413
    review of, 413–421
      consultation with other clinicians, 415, 418
      evaluation requirements, 415
      informed consent, 418–419
      periodic review, 418
      qualifications of physicians, 419–420
      threshold doses and durations, 420–421
      treatment agreements, 419
      urine drug testing, 415
      use of alternatives to opioids, 414
   using chronic pain outcomes data to improve outcomes, **395–408**
    Affordable Care Act, 398–399
      bundled payment for care improvement services, 398–399
      chronic care management services, 399
    Centers for Medicare and Medicaid Services outcomes and opioid prescription
      programs, 399–401
    health care economics, 396–397
    integrating mobile technology, 405–406
    integration into electronic health records, 404–405
    patient-reported outcome measures, 401
    tracking pain outcomes on a national level, 397–398
    Tri-Institutional Pain Registry, 401–404
    utilizing data to improve efficiency and quality, 397
Pain mini-residency, from the VA and Dept. of Defense, 368–370
Patient-controlled analgesia, for acute pain in the emergency department, 273
Patient-reported outcomes measures, in patients with chronic pain, 401
Perioperative surgical home, management of opioid-tolerant patients in, **287–301**
    definitions, 288–289
      opioid tolerance, 289
      opioid-induced hyperalgesia, 289
      opioids, 288
      perioperative surgical home concept, 288
    intraoperative management, 292–294
      dexmedetomidine, 294
      ketamine, 292–293
      lidocaine infusions, 293
      regional anesthesia and analgesia, 293
    postoperative management, 294–295
      multimodal approach to, 294–295
      oral analgesics and restarting home medications, 295
    preoperative assessment, 289–292
    special considerations for opioid addiction therapy, 295–298
      acute pain management services in, 297–298
      buprenorphine, 296–297
      naltrexone, 297

Peripheral nerve neurolytic blockade, for cancer pain, 331
Persistent postsurgical pain, **303–315**
    analgesia for prevention of, 309–311
        gabapentin, 309–310
        ketamine, 310
        multimodal, 311
        NSAIDs, 309
        pregabalin, 310
        regional anesthesia/neuroaxial anesthesia, 310–311
    common surgical procedures associated with, 304–305
        breast surgery, 304
        postamputation phantom limb pain, 305
        thoracic surgery, 304–305
    genetics/epigenetics of, 306–307
    mechanisms for development of, 305–306
    risk factors for development of, 307–309
Phantom limb pain, postamputation, 305
Physicians, state policies on qualifications of, 419–420
Policies, of states. See State policies.
Polysomnography, in patients with chronic pain and sleep disturbance, 381
Postsurgical pain, persistent. See Persistent postsurgical pain.
Pregabalin, for prevention of persistent postsurgical pain, 310

Q

Quality improvement, using chronic pain outcomes data to improve
    outcomes, **395–408**

R

Radiofrequency ablation, for cancer pain, 334
Regional anesthesia, for prevention of persistent postsurgical pain, 310–311
    intraoperative, in opioid-tolerant patients, 293
Regulatory issues, state policies on pain management, **409–424**
        authoritative model policy templates, 410–411
        guidelines originating in state agencies, 412–413
        review of, 413–421
            consultation with other clinicians, 415, 418
            evaluation requirements, 415
            informed consent, 418–419
            periodic review, 418
            qualifications of physicians, 419–420
            threshold doses and durations, 420–421
            treatment agreements, 419
            urine drug testing, 415
            use of alternatives to opioids, 414
    with opioids for chronic pain, 347–348
        FDA labeling changes, 348
        rescheduling of hydrocodone, 348
        risk evaluation and mitigation strategy programs, 347
        upper dose limits, 347

Research, needed on chronic pain and opioids, 346
   VA Pain Research Working Group, 372
Resting-state networks, in the brain, functional MRI imaging of, 260–261
Risk factors, for persistent postsurgical pain, 307–309

S

SCAN-ECHO program, from the VA and Dept. of Defense, 370
Sleep disturbance, in patients with chronic pain, **379–393**
     assessment of, 381–382
     nonpharmacologic interventions, 382–383
     pharmacotherapy, 383–389
        anticonvulsants, 388
        antidepressants, 386–388
        antipsychotics, 388
        benzodiazepine receptor agonists, 385–386
        nonbenzodiazepine benzodiazepine receptor agonists, 386
        opioid analgesics, 383–385
        over the counter medications, 388–389
Spinal cord stimulation, for cancer pain, 336
State policies, regulating practice of pain management, **409–424**
     authoritative model policy templates, 410–411
     guidelines originating in state agencies, 412–413
     review of, 413–421
        consultation with other clinicians, 415, 418
        evaluation requirements, 415
        informed consent, 418–419
        periodic review, 418
        qualifications of physicians, 419–420
        threshold doses and durations, 420–421
        treatment agreements, 419
        urine drug testing, 415
        use of alternatives to opioids, 414
Stepped care, for pain in veterans, 365–368
Stratification Tool for Opioid Risk Management (STORM), from the VA and
   Dept. of Defense, 371
Superior hypogastric plexus neurolysis, for cancer pain, 328–329
Surgery. *See* Perioperative surgical home.
Surgical pain, postoperative. *See* Persistent postsurgical pain.

T

Thoracic surgery, persistent postsurgical pain after, 304–305
Tolerance, opioid, in preoperative assessment, 291
Tri-Institutional Pain Registry, 401–404
Trigeminal neurolysis, for cancer pain, 332–334

U

Urine drug testing, state policies on, 415

V

Vertebral augmentation, for cancer pain, 324
    complications, 324
    contraindications, 324
    indications, 324
    outcomes, 324
Veterans, advancing the pain agenda in, **357–378**
    pain as a public health problem, 357–359
    pain in military personnel and veterans, 359–360
    prevention and reversal of pain chronification, 360–362
    providing education and training, 368–371
    stepped-care approach, 365–368
    structural challenges, 362–365
    VA pain research, 372
Veterans Health Administration, pain programs developed with the Department of Defense, 368–371
    Academic Detailing Service, 371
    Joint Pain Education Project, 368
    Opioid Therapy Risk Report, 371
    Opioids Safety Initiative, 370–371
    Pain Management Nursing Work Group, 371
    Pain Mini-Residency, 368, 370
    Pain Research Working Group, 372
    Pain SCAN-ECHO program, 370
    Stratification Tool for Opioid Risk Management (STORM), 371
    Tiered Acupuncture Training Across Clinical Settings, 368